Convenient Care Clinics

Joshua Riff, MD, MBA, FACEP, is one of the original contributors to the field of convenient care medicine. He pioneered the use of evidence-based medicine and electronic medical records in the retail clinic environment using templates and order sets to drive standardization of care. He attended medical school and received his MBA from Tufts University in conjunction with Brandeis University. After medical school, he attended Johns Hopkins Hospital where he completed his residency in emergency medicine. After practicing emergency medicine in Tucson for 3 years, he moved to Minneapolis to join the retail revolution. While in Minneapolis, he served as Target Clinic's first medical director and later as Target's chief medical director, where he had responsibilities for health care quality and safety for Target's 1,700 pharmacies and 44 clinics. He continued serving the retail industry at WellPoint, where he was the vice president of Retail Clinical Strategy. At WellPoint, he built strategies around onsite and near-site clinics to serve WellPoint's 35 million members. Dr. Riff has given over 100 speeches and lectures with topics ranging from retail clinics to health well-being and to work–life balance. He serves on various boards and committees including the Institute of Medicine, Lifetime Fitness Medical Advisory Board, Institute for Clinical Systems Improvement, and the Retail Clinician Advisory Board. He practices emergency medicine at United Hospital in St Paul, MN, and works at Target Corporation as their medical director and director of well-being.

Sandra F. Ryan, MSN, RN, CPNP, FCPP, FAANP, the first chief nurse practitioner (NP) officer in the convenient care industry, is a founding officer at Take Care Health Systems. She currently leads 1,300 NPs and PAs who practice at Take Care Clinics; walk-in clinics at 360 Walgreens drugstores in 19 states. There, she oversees clinical and operational leadership while working closely with Walgreens chief medical officer in clinical governance, research, and quality initiatives. Ryan has also played an integral role in the development and implementation of integrated technology, quality assurance programs, and evidenced-based guidelines to create a consistent patient-focused experience for those who seek treatment at Take Care Clinics. In addition, Ryan serves as chair of the Clinical Advisory Board of the Convenient Care Association (CCA), where she was instrumental in developing the CCA's Quality and Safety Standards and implementing a third-party certification process for these standards. To address the educational needs of NPs in convenient care, Ryan orchestrated the first Retail Clinician Education Congress, fostering camaraderie and support within the NP community for this emerging model of health care. Ryan has over 25 years of nursing and leadership experience in various clinical, management, and leadership settings. Her experiences as a highly decorated Air Force nurse corps officer include working as a clinician, charge nurse, and director of ambulatory services in inpatient and outpatient settings. Ryan is a recipient of the Nancy Sharp Cutting Edge Award, given by the American College of Nurse Practitioners, and the CARE Leadership Award for contributions to NP practice in the convenient care industry. She is a 2011 Robert Wood Johnson Executive Nurse Fellow and a fellow of the Philadelphia College of Physicians.

Tine Hansen-Turton, MGA, JD, FCPP, FAAN—known as a "systems changer"—is founding executive director/CEO of the Convenient Care Association (CCA) in Philadelphia: a national for-profit trade association of 1,500 (spring 2013) emerging private-sector-based retail clinics that provide basic primary health care to over 20 million people nationally. She also serves as chief strategy officer for Public Health Management Corporation, a nonprofit public health institute, where she oversees half of the organization and leads partnership development around new and emerging business opportunities, and CEO of the National Nursing Centers Consortium, where she oversees the growth and development of 500+ nurse-managed health centers, serving more than 2.5 million clients.

Tine is an adjunct faculty, University of Pennsylvania Fels Institute of Government, Temple University School of Law, and LaSalle University. She writes and publishes for many peer-review professional health care and legal journals and is a regular presenter at national health care conferences. She is a coauthor of *Community and Nurse-Managed Health Centers: Getting Them Started and Keeping Them Going, Nurse-Managed Wellness Centers: Developing and Maintaining Your Center,* both published by Springer Publishing Company, and *Conversations With Leaders,* published by Sigma Theta Tau International. She recently cofounded a volunteer-driven web-based regional journal, *Philadelphia Social Innovations Journal,* which highlights social innovators and innovations in the Philadelphia region. Hansen-Turton has received several recognitions, including the prestigious Eisenhower Fellowship, *Philadelphia Business Journal* 40 under 40 Leadership Award, Philadelphia Connector, and the American Express NextGen Fellow. Tine received her BA from Slippery Rock University, her master's in Government Administration from University of Pennsylvania Fels Institute, and her juris doctor from Temple University Beasley School of Law.

MANAGING EDITOR

Caroline G. Ridgway, JD, worked as the policy and communications director for the Convenient Care Association (CCA), the national trade organization representing the retail-based convenient care clinic industry, for more than 5 years, where she was responsible for coordinating the government affairs and policy initiatives of the association and its members, for executing communications outreach and strategies, and for developing and advancing the overall strategic vision of the CCA. With CCA, Caroline was regularly featured around the country as a conference presenter about policy issues related to the retail-based health care industry, and frequently testified in front of state legislative and regulatory committees. Caroline also severed as the managing editor for the *Philadelphia Social Innovations Journal,* an academic journal focused on promoting social innovation and entrepreneurship in and around the Philadelphia region. Caroline received her BA in psychology with a concentration in neural and behavioral sciences from Haverford College and her JD from Temple University Beasley School of Law.

Convenient Care Clinics

The Essential Guide to Retail Clinics for Clinicians, Managers, and Educators

Joshua Riff, MD, MBA, FACEP

Sandra F. Ryan, MSN, RN, CPNP, FCPP, FAANP

Tine Hansen-Turton, MGA, JD, FCCP, FAAN

Editors

Caroline G. Ridgway, JD
Managing Editor

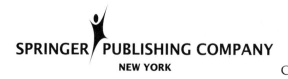

SPRINGER PUBLISHING COMPANY
NEW YORK

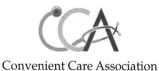

Convenient Care Association

Springer Publishing Company, LLC
11 West 42nd Street
New York, NY 10036
www.springerpub.com

Acquisitions Editor: Margaret Zuccarini
Composition: diacriTech

ISBN: 978-0-8261-2126-4
e-book ISBN: 978-0-8261-2127-1

13 14 15 16 / 5 4 3 2 1

The author and the publisher of this Work have made every effort to use sources believed to be reliable to provide information that is accurate and compatible with the standards generally accepted at the time of publication. Because medical science is continually advancing, our knowledge base continues to expand. Therefore, as new information becomes available, changes in procedures and drug dosages become necessary. We recommend that the reader always consult current research and specific institutional policies and formularies before performing any clinical procedure or prescribing any drug. The author and publisher shall not be liable for any special, consequential, or exemplary damages resulting, in whole or in part, from the readers' use of, or reliance on, the information contained in this book. The publisher has no responsibility for the persistence or accuracy of URLs for external or third-party Internet websites referred to in this publication and does not guarantee that any content on such websites is, or will remain, accurate or appropriate.

Library of Congress Cataloging-in-Publication Data

Convenient care clinics: the essential guide to retail clinics for clinicians, managers, and educators / Joshua Riff, MD, MBA, FACEP, Sandra F. Ryan, MSN, RN, CPNP, FCPP, FAANP, Tine Hansen-Turton, MGA, JD, FCCP, FAAN, editors; Caroline G. Ridgway, JD, managing editor.
    pages cm
Includes bibliographical references and index.
ISBN 978-0-8261-2126-4
1. Ambulatory medical care—United States. 2. Emergency medical services—United States. 3. Integrated delivery of health care—United States. 4. Health facilities, Proprietary—United States. I. Riff, Joshua, editor of compilation. II. Ryan, Sandra F., editor of compilation. III. Hansen-Turton, Tine, editor of compilation. IV. Ridgway, Caroline G., editor of compilation.
RA395.A3C737 2013
362.18—dc23
                                                2013006458

Printed in the United States of America by Bang Printing.

Contents

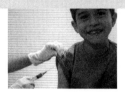

Contributors   *ix*
Foreword by Susan B. Hassmiller, PhD, RN, FAAN   *xi*
Preface   *xiii*

1. The Future of Accessible, Affordable, Quality Health Care   *1*
   Tine Hansen-Turton and Caroline G. Ridgway

PART I   CLINICAL CHAPTERS

2. Approach to the Convenient Care Clinic Patient With Ear Pain   *11*
   Sandra F. Ryan and Mark R. Nielsen

3. Red Eye and Other Eye Complaints   *23*
   Tracey J. Kniess and Sandra F. Ryan

4. Approach to the Patient With a Sore Throat   *39*
   Lynette Sullivan and Joshua Riff

5. Sinusitis   *51*
   Nia Valentine and Samuel N. Grief

6. Cough and Upper Respiratory Tract Infections   *61*
   Joshua Riff and Sandra F. Ryan

7. Dysuria and Urinary Complaints   *73*
   Sangeetha Larsen and Augustine Sohn

8. Rashes   *83*
   Lori Crews and Brian Zelickson

9. Fever   *99*
   Kiley Black

10. Vital Signs: Recognizing and Managing Abnormalities   *111*
    Jill Johnson, Mary C. Homan, and Sandra F. Ryan

11. Sports Physicals: The Preparticipation Physical Evaluation   *121*
    Susan M. Cooley, Elizabeth Perius, and Kevin Ronneberg

12. Specific Populations in the Convenient Care Clinic Setting   *129*
    Tania Celia and Sandra F. Ryan

13. Vaccinations in the Convenient Care Clinic   *137*
    Barbara Spychalla and Sandra F. Ryan

14. Making Sense of the Over-the-Counter Market   *143*
    Elliott M. Sogol

15. Strategies to Improve Antibiotic Prescribing in Convenient Care   *153*
    Rebecca M. Roberts, Lauri A. Hicks, and Joshua Riff

PART II   THE BUSINESS OF CONVENIENT CARE CLINICS

16. Building and Marketing a Retail Clinic   *161*
    Mary Kate Scott

17. Measuring Customer Satisfaction—Understanding the Consumer
    Mindset   *171*
    Paul H. Keckley

18. The Dollars and Cents of Running a Clinic   *179*
    Webster F. Golinkin and Danielle Barrera

19. Research and Quality, Cost, and Access   *187*
    Caroline G. Ridgway

20. Quality Metrics and Initiatives in the Clinic Setting   *193*
    Janice M. Miller and David B. Nash

21. Collaboration and Partnership in the Convenient Care Setting   *201*
    William D. Wright and Eileen Stellefson Myers

22. The Future of Convenient Care Clinics and Health Care Reform   *207*
    Jason Hwang

Appendix: Profiles of Clinic Operators   217
References   231
Index   243

Contributors

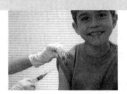

Danielle Barrera
Chief Operating Officer
RediClinic
Houston, TX

Kiley Black, RN, CNP
Manager, Clinics Standards and
    Medical Education
Target Corporation
Minneapolis, MN

Tania Celia, MSN, FNP
Clinical Educator
Take Care Health Systems
Conshohocken, PA

Susan M. Cooley, PhD, RN, CPNP
VP Clinical Services
RediClinic
Houston, TX

Lori Crews, MSN, FNP
Director of Site Operations
Take Care Health Systems
Conshohocken, PA

Webster F. Golinkin
Chief Executive Officer
RediClinic
Houston, TX

Samuel N. Grief, MD, FCFP
Associate Professor, Clinical Family
    Medicine
University of Illinois at Chicago
Chicago, IL

Lauri A. Hicks, DO
Medical Epidemiologist
Centers for Disease Control and
    Prevention
Atlanta, GA

Mary C. Homan, MD, MPH
Physician, Family Medicine
Fairview Health Services
Rosemount, MN

Jason Hwang, MD, MBA
Founder
Innosight Institute
San Mateo, CA

**Jill Johnson, DNP, APRN, FNP-BC,
    CCRN, CEN, CFRN**
Market Manager, Louisville
Take Care Health Systems
Conshohocken, PA

Paul H. Keckley, PhD
Executive Director
Deloitte Center for Health
    Solutions
Washington, DC

**Tracey J. Kniess, DNP, CRNP,
    FNP-BC**
Senior Manager, Clinical
    Education
Take Care Health Systems
Conshohocken, PA

Sangeetha Larsen, PA-C
Physician Assistant
Target Clinic
Minneapolis, MN

Janice M. Miller, DNP, CRNP, CDE
Assistant Professor and Program
  Coordinator, Adult/Gerontology
  Nurse Practitioner Program
Jefferson School of Nursing,
  Thomas Jefferson University
Philadelphia, PA

Eileen Stellefson Myers, MPH, RD
Senior Director, Healthcare Alliances
  and Health Management
The Little Clinic, LLC
Nashville, TN

David B. Nash, MD, MBA
Dean
Jefferson School of Population
  Health
Philadelphia, PA

Mark R. Nielsen, MD
Physician, Internal Medicine
Fairview Health Services
Bloomington, MN

Elizabeth Perius, PhD, RN, ENP
Nurse Practitioner
RediClinic
Houston, TX

Rebecca M. Roberts, MS
Public Health Specialist
Centers for Disease Control and
  Prevention
Atlanta, GA

Kevin Ronneberg, MD
Associate Medical Director
Target Corporation
Minneapolis, MN

Mary Kate Scott
Principal
Scott & Company, Inc.
Hartland, ME

**Elliott M. Sogol, PhD, RPh,
  FAPhA**
Professional Services
Target Corporation
Minneapolis, MN

Augustine Sohn, MD, MPH
Assistant Professor, Clinical Family
  Medicine
College of Medicine, University of
  Illinois at Chicago
Chicago, IL

**Barbara Spychalla, MSN,
  FNP-BC**
Nurse Practitioner
Take Care Health Systems
Conshohocken, PA

**Lynette Sullivan, ARNP, FNP-C,
  MSN, BSN**
Family Nurse Practitioner
Take Care Health Systems
Conshohocken, PA

Nia Valentine, MS, CRNP-F
Executive Team Leader – Clinic
Target Clinic
Minneapolis, MN

William D. Wright, JD, MTS
Chief Legal Officer
The Little Clinic, LLC
Nashville, TN

Brian Zelickson, MD
Zel Skin and Laser Specialists
Associate Professor of Dermatology,
  University of Minnesota
Minneapolis, MN

Foreword

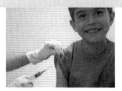

One Thursday night, a number of years ago, my mother came down with an excruciating earache. She couldn't sleep. Her doctor's office was closed; hence, I drove her to the emergency room. We waited for 3 hours for a doctor to spend 2 minutes examining her ear and prescribe her an antibiotic to treat what she thought was an ear infection. We returned home, but her pain did not diminish that night or the next.

After 3 days, I thought of the convenient care clinic (CCC) in the pharmacy in our town. I took my mother to the clinic on a Sunday morning. The nurse who saw my mother introduced herself and asked what had happened. My mother explained her story, and the nurse asked her whether she had stuck anything in her ear. My mother remembered that she had inserted a bobby pin in her ear to stop the ear from itching. The nurse realized that my mother was suffering from an inflammation from scratching her inner ear with the bobby pin. She gave my mother some anti-inflammatory ear drops and advised her not to stick bobby pins in her ear again. Two days later, a card arrived in our mailbox from the nurse who had treated my mother, saying that she was glad she had stopped by and to call if her ear still hurt. That's when I became a strong supporter of CCCs. The personalized and attentive care that my mother received offered a glimpse of how nurses could be better utilized to improve patient care.

And we desperately need to improve patient care. Our health care system faces enormous challenges. In 2014, an additional 32 million Americans will receive health insurance, and we need to ensure that enough primary care providers will be available to treat them. Our population is aging, and getting sicker because of more chronic health conditions. Health care disparities continue to plague our system. Too many people die from medical errors, and costs continue to skyrocket. In 2010, the United States spent $2.6 trillion on health care, or 17.6% of GDP, significantly more than any other country and more than twice as much as relatively rich European countries such as France, Sweden, and the United Kingdom. Yet our quality lags behind other nations (OECD, 2012). The emergency room is one of the most expensive settings in which to treat patients (Agency for Healthcare Research and Quality [AHRQ], 2011). That's why it's crucial that our country find ways to keep patients out of the emergency room except for true emergencies. We need to do a better job managing chronic illnesses, so that patients do not rely on the emergency room and hospital for care. The challenges are daunting, and we need innovative solutions to address our nation's most pressing health care challenges—access, quality, and cost.

One of the Institute of Medicine (IOM) recommendations calls for private and public funders, health care organizations, nursing education programs, and nursing associations to expand opportunities for nurses to lead and manage collaborative efforts with physicians and other members of the health care team. CCCs are a perfect example of an innovative, patient-centered care model that should be diffused widely—they are critical to improving access to care, and they save costs by enabling people with minor ailments to get treated without going to the emergency room. CCCs provide "just in time" access to help people get the care they need when they need it. They also treat people in the communities where they live, learn, work, and play.

I am heartened that *Convenient Care Clinics: The Essential Guide to Retail Clinics for Clinicians, Managers, and Educators* will be used to expose students to CCCs as an innovative solution that is helping to improve health care. I hope this book will inspire more practitioners to work at CCCs and to develop other innovative businesses to improve health and health care. We need greater collaboration among health professionals to improve patient care. I also hope that nurse practitioners and physician assistants who work at CCCs will use this book as a valuable resource.

I knew from my first visit with my mother that CCCs represented the future of health care. They offer expanded access and quality services for patients at moderate cost. In addition, they enable nurse practitioners and physician assistants to practice to the full extent of their education and training while freeing physicians to treat more complex patients. This book will serve as a valuable resource in ensuring that our future nurse practitioners, physician assistants, and physicians are well versed in the benefits of convenient care clinics.

For more information about the Campaign for Action and to find out how you can become involved in your state, visit the Campaign's website at http://campaignforaction.org.

Susan B. Hassmiller, PhD, RN, FAAN
Senior Adviser for Nursing
Robert Wood Johnson Foundation

Preface

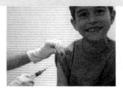

The advent and rise of the convenient care industry directly reflects a growing demand for consumer-driven health care and an unmet need for health care access in our country. Built on the foundations of providing easily accessible, affordable, high-quality health care, retail-based convenient care clinics (CCCs) represent an innovative, "disruptive" change that has revolutionized health care access and delivery in the United States. In about a decade, the industry has expanded from a few clinics to approximately 1,400 clinics in 39 states and growing.

The three of us are incredibly proud to have been part of the inception and growth of a new industry that has changed health care as we know it. Together with our colleagues around the country, we created an unparalleled patient experience and made health care costs, quality scores, and wait times transparent and easily accessible to patients. We set new expectations for how patients could access clinicians and how evidence-based medicine could be delivered consistently across the country on a large scale. More importantly, CCCs have been able to become part of the solution and a complement to the current health care system. Partnerships and relationships are continuously forming between convenient care operators and other key stakeholders to meet the needs of patients. CCCs are being seen as a vital part of the health care continuum.

As far as this industry has come in a decade's time, we are cognizant that there is work yet to be done. As convenient care continues to evolve to meet the needs of the communities it serves, it will be important to strengthen and deepen the relationships the clinics have with the health care community as a whole. Critical to the future vitality of our health care system will be a dual focus on workforce development and support and on applying a collaborative and inclusive perspective to patient care. It is in that spirit that convenient care has emerged and grown and in which this book was written.

Everyone who works in this industry has direct insight into the health care problems that exist today, understands the future needs of patients, and has made a decision to be part of a movement that will be part of the solution to our health care crisis for decades to come. Nationally, there is a compelling need for access to acute, episodic care, which has been the clinical backbone of the convenient care industry since its founding. CCC operators have also identified and responded to increasing demand for preventive care, wellness support, and assistance with diagnosis and management of chronic illness. Strong patient satisfaction ratings and quality indicators demonstrate that the clinics are filling a void in care and meaningfully complementing existing care delivery.

A successful future for our national health care delivery system will require committed efforts from many stakeholders, including entrepreneurs, administrators, educators, retailers, and others, supporting and buffering providers' daily efforts. Being innovative, challenging the status quo, and continuing to focus on quality outcomes that will improve the health of our nation should be the ongoing charge for all of us.

NOTE TO READERS

In many chapters recommended drugs and dosages are provided. With time and regional variation these are subject to change. Please use an up-to-date reference when choosing medication and dosage.

Joshua Riff, MD, MBA, FACEP
Sandra F. Ryan, MSN, RN, CPNP, FCPP, FAANP
Tine Hansen-Turton, MGA, JD, FCCP, FAAN

1

The Future of Accessible, Affordable, Quality Health Care

TINE HANSEN-TURTON AND CAROLINE G. RIDGWAY

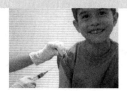

Only in the past decade has convenient care evolved from nothing more than an intriguing idea to a novel but untested business model to an established and viable industry with a tangible impact on national health care.

This chapter examines the history and evolution of the convenient care industry (CCI), its model and popularity, and why it works.

HISTORY

Health care driven by the needs of consumers is the bedrock of the CCI. Since their inception, the retail-based convenient care clinics (CCCs) have been consumer favorites; they are known for providing affordable, accessible, quality health care to consumers who would typically have to wait hours, days, or even weeks for basic primary care.

Early on, CCCs became media favorites because they challenged the status quo in health care delivery. The clinics raised concerns from the medical establishment, resulting in articles that showed a medical community at odds with innovation and with new market entrants.

However, despite opposing views, reporters have consistently written about the expectation that retail health clinics will "profoundly affect health care delivery by providing an alternative site for basic medical care" (Malvey & Fottler, 2006). CCCs have been called a "disruptive innovation" by Harvard University professor and *New York Times* best-selling author Clayton Christensen, because they represent a new interpretation of an old and user-unfriendly system; CCCs are consumer driven and respond to patients who "are frustrated with the conventional health care delivery system," which is known for providing inadequate access to basic health care services when people need them the most (Christensen, Grossman, & Hwang, 2009).

The first CCC, operated by QuickMedx (which later became MinuteClinic, now owned by CVS), opened its doors in 2000 in the Minneapolis–St. Paul area. The founders of the clinic recognized that the existing primary care infrastructure was not meeting patients' basic health care needs. From 2000 to 2006, new market entrants began to open clinics in retail settings with financial backing from venture capital companies. Today, there are multiple organizations (private, nonprofit, and hospitals) across the country that manage CCCs. Some of the current leading clinic operators include MinuteClinic, owned and operated by CVS Caremark; Take Care Health Systems, owned and operated by Walgreen Co.; The Little Clinic, owned and operated by Kroger; Target; RediClinic; and Lindora; as well as major hospitals across the country. Walmart serves as a landlord for a number of CCCs, and, more recently, health insurers are operating their own CCCs.

ROLE OF NONPHYSICIAN PROVIDERS IN PRIMARY CARE

The CCI could not have expanded without a revolution in primary care, which started in 1965 with the establishment of two new primary care provider groups, nurse practitioners (NPs), and physician assistants (PAs): NPs remain the largest single group of providers working in the CCI.

Nurse-managed care is not new to health care; in fact, nursing practices over the years sprang up in fields where physicians had not yet established footholds, for example, nurse midwifery and rural health (Mezey, McGivern, Sullivan-Marx, & Greenberg, 2003). After World War II, nursing education took off; nurses who had practiced in the war could pursue advanced education through the G.I. Bill and began to work in communities throughout the United States (Mezey et al., 2003). In the 1960s, when Medicare and Medicaid legislation passed, there was a new demand for services, and it became apparent that there was an inadequate supply of physicians to meet this growing demand. This shortage enabled both the expansion of other professions, like nursing, into primary care and the development of new types of providers, such as NPs (Mezey et al., 2003). The first NP program was established at the University of Colorado in 1965 by nursing professor Loretta Ford and pediatrician Henry Silver (Mezey et al., 2003). Other programs were quickly established, and the degree was popular from the start, attracting nurses to pursue advanced degrees. In parallel, at Duke University in 1965, Dr. Eugene Stead started the nation's first PA program, initially deployed in the military but eventually taking off at universities across the United States (Vorvick, 2011).

Both the NP and PA roles have grown a great deal since the mid-1980s, receiving a boost in 1994 when the Institute of Medicine's Committee on the Future of Primary Care broadly defined primary care as "the provision of integrated, accessible health care services by clinicians who are accountable for addressing a large majority of personal health care needs, developing a sustained partnership with patients, and practicing in the context of family and community" (Donaldson, Yordy, & Vanselow, 1994). As of 2010, the Agency for Healthcare Research and Quality estimated that there were more than 106,000 practicing NPs and 70,000 practicing PAs (http://www.ahrq.gov/research/pcwork2.htm).

In 2012, more than 5,000 NPs and PAs are working in the CCI, and the need will only grow as the industry evolves and expands.

THE RETAIL-BASED CCC MODEL

The CCC model is still evolving based on consumer needs and as health care reform unfolds. During the first stage of the industry (2000–2005), only a very limited number of illnesses were treated in the clinics. For example, QuickMedx (now MinuteClinic) treated only seven conditions: strep throat; mononucleosis; flu; pregnancy testing; and bladder, ear, and sinus infections. The clinics were offered as cost-effective alternatives to basic, episodic care and as a way to keep patients out of expensive emergency rooms for basic care. QuickMedx founders Rick Krieger and Douglas Smith wanted to establish a model of care delivery that permitted patients with relatively simple medical needs to receive efficient, effective treatment without the long delays and high costs associated with the traditional health care system. The first clinics that opened accepted only cash for services, and other market entrants modeled themselves after QuickMedx. However, it soon became clear that additional services could be added to the menu and that the cash model was limiting the clinics' ability to grow and scale.

It was apparent early on that consumers supported the CCC model. Mothers with children were early adopters of convenient care, recognizing its value in providing basic care when children's pediatricians were not available or on weekends or evenings when traditional primary care offices are closed. Early on, consumers encouraged their employers and insurance providers to sign on with the clinics. Today, all clinic operators accept health insurance, and some insurers even provide incentives for their enrollees to use the clinics for nonemergent care. Furthermore, the scope of services has significantly expanded based on consumer needs and feedback and today includes a broader range of acute care, preventive services, and some chronic disease management, usually in partnership with hospitals.

CCC Description

CCCs are usually located in retail locations, such as drugstores, food stores, and other retail settings with pharmacies. Because of these retail locations, CCCs provide easy accessibility and are convenient for patients, who can get any needed prescriptions filled on site. The clinics range in size from one examination room to multiple, with sinks and examination tables. The clinics generally occupy 500 square feet and are outfitted with all the necessities of an outpatient health care office. Federal laws require that owners and operators of the clinics rent retail space at fair market value as assessed by an appraiser. The providers, like NPs and PAs, who staff the CCCs usually work for the operators of the clinics and have a collegial relationship with the pharmacy staff of the retail setting. Given their retail location, most of the clinics are open 7 days a week, 12 hours a day during the week, and 8 hours on weekends; these hours are generally more convenient than those of traditional doctors and primary care providers. Nearly half of CCC visits take place on weekends and during weekday hours when primary care offices are typically closed, reflecting their convenience and consumer focus. Most of the clinics see patients 18 months of age and older, and visits generally take 15 to 25 minutes for diagnosis and treatment. Clinic providers diagnose, treat, and write prescriptions for common illnesses such as strep throat; pinkeye; and infections of the ears, nose, throat, and bladder. They also provide vaccinations for flu, pneumonia, pertussis, and hepatitis, among others. Furthermore, they treat minor wounds, abrasions, joint sprains, and skin conditions such as poison ivy, ringworm, and acne. In addition, they offer routine lab tests and provide a wide range of wellness services, including sports and camp physicals, smoking cessation, TB testing, and chronic disease monitoring, and related services for those with diabetes, high cholesterol, high blood pressure, and asthma.

The CCI believes strongly in the transparency of medical costs. All CCC operators post their services and costs, whether visibly at the clinic, on the clinic's website, or through a brochure or other mechanism, and the basic cash cost for a visit to a CCC averages $75 (Thygeson, Van Vorst, Maciosek, & Solberg, 2008).

Since the industry's inception, the clinics have been primarily staffed by NPs and to a lesser extent by PAs as well; physicians collaborate with the clinics' providers as needed and as required by state law and regulation. In addition to delivering the patient care in the clinics, clinic providers typically handle some or most of the administrative functions. Some clinics also have medical assistants who aid the provider and help with patient flow. Electronic health records (EHRs) and other technology are used to enhance the patient experience and, with patient consent, ensure coordination and continuity of care with their medical home and primary care providers. All clinics have written guidelines and established protocols that the providers use to assist with decision making and to ensure the highest level of patient care and satisfaction.

The typical visit to a CCC will start with patient registration, in most cases using a touch-screen computer terminal similar to an airline self-check-in kiosk. The computer will ask for basic demographic information and the reason for the visit, and this sign-in process initiates the patient's personal health record. For those who need help, there is usually assistance in the store or a phone number to reach technical assistance. Information captured at the kiosk is then transmitted electronically to a computer terminal inside the treatment room, where a provider is notified of a patient waiting to be seen. Once the patient is escorted to the examination room, the provider validates the information provided at check-in and enters additional information about symptoms, conditions, and any pertinent medical history. To determine diagnosis and treatment, providers perform Clinical Laboratory Improvement Act (CLIA)-waived lab tests and write prescriptions that can be transmitted electronically to the store pharmacy or any other location that accepts e-prescribing. With patients' consent, their visit records are shared with their primary care providers, contributing to continuity of care. With up to 60% of patients using the clinics reporting that they don't have a regular primary care provider, CCCs have become strong partners with local medical communities, referring their patients who don't have a medical home; up to 40% to 50% of people using CCCs also don't have an existing medical home.

Founding of the Industry and the Convenient Care Association

In the summer of 2006, Hal Rosenbluth, founder of Take Care Health Systems, held a summit to which he invited stakeholders to network and make introductions with the idea of shaping the future of the industry. Participants included a cross-section of people: clinic operators, providers, NP leadership, medical and PA representatives, and other stakeholders. Two overarching concerns were the need to ensure that quality was at the forefront of the model and to emphasize that one clinic operator not adhering to quality standards could put the entire nascent industry at risk. One meeting attendee, former secretary of the U.S. Department of Health and Human Services Donna Shalala, suggested that the stakeholders form a more permanent group. Her recommendation was the birth of the CCC trade association, the Convenient Care Association (CCA), which organized with the support of founding members and retail clinic operators Hal Rosenbluth and Webster F. Golinkin and clinic consultant Tine Hansen-Turton.

The CCA was incorporated in October 2006. By that fall, CCA was operational and had begun to focus on implementing the summit recommendations to create a mechanism that would ensure quality. In November 2006, CCA held its first board meeting of the majority of the retail clinic operators at that time and laid out the roadmap to establish quality and safety standards for the industry. The goal was to have standards approved in spring 2007 and a certification program that would ensure the highest quality standards. (CCA certification is described in a later chapter.)

Since its inception, the CCA has positioned itself as a nationally recognized organization. Accomplishments to date include developing and adopting industry quality and safety standards, including implementing third-party certification; advocating successfully against legislation and regulations that would reduce consumer access to the kind of high-quality, affordable health care that CCCs provide; providing continuing education to thousands of CCC practitioners; establishing CCA as a reliable media source; and creating National Convenient Care Clinic Week.

The years 2006 and 2007 were marked with industry acquisitions. In July 2006, CVS Caremark announced that it would acquire Minneapolis-based MinuteClinic (formerly known as QuickMedx) and establish MinuteClinic as a wholly owned subsidiary. In May 2007, Walgreen Co. acquired Conshohocken, PA–based Take Care Health Systems. In May 2008, the Kroger Co. and The Little Clinic announced a partnership whereby Kroger became a shareholder, and in April 2010, Kroger bought the outstanding shares in The Little Clinic and became the owner of the company.

The onset of the recession in 2008 presented significant challenges for the CCI. The nascence of the industry and the low profit margins associated with the business model contributed to the closing of some of the smaller industry operators. However, this period also represented an opportunity for existing providers to expand clinic services and fine tune operations, resulting in a stronger industry today, with 1,400 clinics and growing.

Initial Challenges From the Medical Establishment and Public Skepticism

In light of the small number of clinics nationally and questions about the viability of the business model, the founding of the CCA was initially considered premature. However, it proved prescient when industry opponents—in particular, national medical organizations—promptly issued the first formal challenges to convenient care.

The American Medical Association (AMA), American Academy of Family Physicians (AAFP), and American Academy of Pediatrics (AAP) were the first to publicly question retail-based convenient care. Initial opposition to the convenient care model centered on three specific issues: quality of care, continuity of care, and conflict of interest owing to the ownership model of the clinics. Allegations of poor quality intimated that a health care practice without regular on-site physician oversight, and that was primarily under the day-to-day direction of NPs and PAs, could not meet adequate quality standards and ensure care outcomes. As to continuity of care, opponents of convenient care posited that a model of care based largely around acute, episodic interactions with patients would by default miss key longitudinal care opportunities, such as preventive health counseling and vaccinations. The conflict-of-interest argument supposed that a health care practice owned by and situated inside a for-profit retail setting would be unable to provide objective, focused health care services. For instance, it was suggested that the clinics would overprescribe antibiotics and other unneeded medications simply to drive business to the retail host's co-located pharmacy.

Initial public awareness of and support for convenient care was also middling. Early CCC operators had presumed that overall demand for access and word of mouth would be sufficient to drive increased patient traffic, but it soon became evident that more concerted marketing efforts would be required to drive the volume of patient visits needed to sustain the business. Today, however, there is both high acceptance of the clinics and high patient satisfaction.

Increasing Involvement With and From Hospitals
and Health Systems

As the CCI has grown and evolved, one of the most striking changes over time has been the vastly increased involvement of health systems. Today, all the major operators have strategic partnerships with hospitals for referrals, as well as service expansion opportunities like chronic disease management and maintenance. Although several health systems were very early adopters of retail-based health care and were among the founding members of the CCA (e.g., Aurora, Geisinger, and Sutter), the majority of the first CCC operators were private corporations. In recent years, however, a large number of health systems have entered into the retail-based health care space in one of two main capacities: as direct operators of CCCs in partnership with retail host stores, or as partners with another CCC operator, providing collaborative physicians and allowing for a more streamlined transition of patient care from episodic to ongoing.

COMMITMENTS TO QUALITY

From the outset, the CCI, with the leadership of the CCA, made a strong commitment to quality of care. One of the first steps taken by the CCA was to establish a set of quality and safety standards to which all members would be required to adhere.

The establishment of quality standards for the industry was key to ensure the safety and delivery of the highest quality care in CCCs. Specifically, industry leaders and operators agreed to support the following industry-wide, consumer-driven patient care performance standards:

- Use of national evidence-based guidelines for each condition treated
- Measurably high patient satisfaction
- Tracked set of minimum standards for wait times
- Tracked numbers of patient visits to the clinic
- A health care provider referral system in all markets, allowing for timely treatment of conditions beyond the center's scope of practice
- Tracked cost transparency to patients
- Adherence to OSHA (Occupational Safety & Health Administration) and CLIA standards
- Established quality monitoring and improvement programs
- Established corporate compliance programs
- Established emergency response plans and emergency equipment available at each site
- Established post-visit access plans
- Available discharge instructions and educational materials for each patient
- Established minimum age for pediatric patients
- EHR use with evidence-based protocols from key national organizations

Mechanisms for monitoring patient-driven performance standards were implemented and tracked across the industry. To ensure quality outcomes, visit records were to be shared with the patient and the patient's provider(s) following the Health Insurance Portability and Accountability Act guidelines. The industry, in an effort to integrate care within the medical community, also recommended that all health care providers aspire to the following patient-centric practices:

- Use of EHRs
- Ability to take convenient care referrals within 24 hours
- Ability to send follow-up information back to the CCC for patients who were referred out
- Ability to accept new primary care patients within 2 to 3 weeks (approximately 20% to 30% of patients coming to a CCC require a medical home)
- Collaborative, patient-centered, evidence-based health care

A clinical advisory board consisting of representatives of both clinic operators and national medical, nursing, and accrediting organizations was responsible for developing the quality and safety standards. In 2010, the CCA revised the standards to reflect maturation in the industry.

Before the quality and safety standards have been developed, CCA leadership recognized the importance of providing all its members with an accessible path to third-party certification. Although some clinic were operators elected early on to pursue accreditation with The Joint Commission, the CCA entered into a partnership with Jefferson Medical College to administer a certification developed specifically for its members. The certification has been well received and has been a useful tool for clinic operators negotiating contracts with third-party payers.

Quality care and quality assurance are critical to the long-term survival of the CCI. Thus, at most CCCs, standardized protocols assist NPs in clinical decision making. These protocols are guidelines—they are not intended to replace the critical thinking and clinical judgment of the provider, but only to enhance and assist in the decision-making process. The leading CCCs' practices are grounded in evidence-based medicine and guidelines published by major medical bodies such as the AAP and AAFP. The clinics have incorporated rigorous quality assessments into their evaluative structures, including both internal and external reviews such as formal chart review by collaborating physicians and peer review by providers with additional standard coding auditing. Provider credentialing and thorough work history are established, as is a process for ensuring that those working in this independent role have adequate experience. CCCs strive to establish a referral base with physicians and other health care providers in the best interest of their patients, their providers, and the continuity of health care within the medical community. The CCI adheres to all state regulations regarding practice issues for the advance practice nurse and PA.

FUTURE DIRECTIONS

Over time, the scope of services offered in the convenient care setting has steadily expanded, while staying within a range of treatments that can be carried out in 15 to 20 minutes and that don't require substantial or invasive diagnostic testing. Retail-based CCCs have evolved at a time when our health care system is floundering. The focus of the CCI is quality, convenience, and consumer choice. CCCs have established standards, employ competent professional primary care providers, and use ongoing quality improvement mechanisms, including the incorporation of evidence-based practices in patient care. Health care delivery systems are changing in multifaceted ways and are constantly in flux. CCCs have identified the need for change and are filling a niche by moving to bridge the chasm between a failing health care system and a rising new model that offers high-quality, cost-effective, and timely health care.

With the Supreme Court's summer 2012 decision to uphold the Affordable Care Act, the need for accessible, affordable, quality health care has never been greater. Equally great is the value proposition of the retail-based CCC model of care, so the industry is poised for future success.

Approach to the Convenient Care Clinic Patient With Ear Pain

SANDRA F. RYAN AND
MARK R. NIELSEN

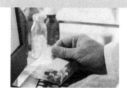

Otalgia, or ear pain, is a common presenting complaint in the convenient care clinical setting. The origin of otalgia may be either primary (otogenic) or secondary (referred) in nature. In children, ear pain often tends to be due to primary ear disease, with secondary causes being more common in adults. This chapter reviews some of the common causes of primary and secondary otalgia.

Case Study: A 28-year-old male presents complaining of right ear pain. He has a sensation of water in the ear, and he cannot hear well. He denies any recent illness or air travel and has no known chronic medical problems. When questioned about possible precipitating events, he reports that he had been water skiing on a lake the day before and had caught a wake wrong and fell to his right, striking his head and shoulder hard against the water. He states that he also noticed some dried blood on his pillow this morning, but hasn't had any further drainage from the right ear. He denies dizziness or vertigo.

On physical examination, he is alert and in no acute distress. His left ear is unremarkable; there is some blood on the floor of the canal of the right ear. The tympanic membrane (TM) shows moderate injection and a large, central, jagged perforation with approximately 30% of the TM absent. The middle-ear space is clean and dry, and the rest of the physical examination is unremarkable.

CLINICAL EVALUATION

Key points to elicit when collecting patient history are onset, location (have the patient point with a finger), radiation, duration, associated symptoms (otologic and systemic), and precipitating events such as a recent upper respiratory infection (URI), flight, trauma, or water exposure. It is also important to determine whether there has been any hearing impairment or discharge.

Another important factor to consider is the patient's age and lifestyle habits. Patients older than 50 and those with prior or current tobacco and/or alcohol use are at greater risk for tumors of the head and neck (Ely, Hansen, & Clark, 2008). Along this line, it is imperative to ask specifically about vocal changes or dysphagia when considering an occult process.

Surgical history is important as well, especially if the patient has had prior ear surgery. Patients who have had ventilation tubes inserted in the past typically have a history of chronic middle-ear infections. In addition, a history of prior mastoidectomy, tympanoplasty, or ossiculoplasty indicates more complication and may call for referral to an ear, nose, and throat (ENT) specialist.

Physical Examination

The examination should start with vital signs, because a high fever is an important red flag in the workup of ear pain. Although low-grade fevers are common with ear infections, a high fever in a toxic-appearing patient can indicate more serious complications such as meningitis or mastoiditis and thus is a cause for concern. Every patient should have an inspection and palpation of the auricle, including the pre- and postauricular areas, noting any discomfort with manipulation as well as noting any lymphadenopathy. Look for signs of trauma and comment if any redness or swelling is present in the external ear. Always perform an external ear exam, and consider otitis externa (OE) if there is pain when pulling on the pinna of the ear or palpation of the tragus.

Next, a full otoscopic examination is necessary to identify any abnormalities of the canal, TM, and middle ear space; cerumen or debris removal may be necessary to complete this assessment. It often helps to start the examination with the "good" ear for comparison. In addition, a gross hearing test (whisper or finger rub) and pneumotoscopy may be helpful (Ely et al., 2008) and should be commented on in the chart.

The problem-focused examination should also include examining the nose and oropharynx and palpation of the head and neck, including the temporomandibular joints (TMJs); this is especially important when the ear examination is normal. With the oral examination, careful attention should be given to the gingiva, teeth, and posterior pharynx as these are frequent sources of secondary otalgia (Ely et al., 2008) with observation to the patient's vocal quality. Also palpate the mastoid bone to rule out a mastoid infection. Commenting on the function of the cranial nerves is also helpful.

DIFFERENTIAL DIAGNOSIS

Primary ear pain is usually caused by one of three conditions: OE, acute otitis media (AOM), and otitis media with effusion. Rare but serious complications of primary ear infections can develop and include mastoiditis, meningitis, and malignant OE. Secondary ear pain (or referred pain) is most likely due to dental processes; however, red flags such as trauma or a history of oral tobacco use can be harbingers of more serious disease.

As noted above, otalgia can be of primary or secondary (referred) origin. Red flags that can help the provider decide when to refer to an ENT specialist include the following:

- Patients with persistent effusion following barotrauma
- Foreign bodies (FBs) that are embedded in the canal or TM or cannot be removed safely
- Patients with herpes zoster with complaint of hearing loss
- Suspected cases of temporal arteritis (ear pain with a tender temporal region in elderly patients, with or without a headache)
- Unexplained, persistent, unilateral ear pain in the adult patient
- Patients with large, acute TM perforations
- Patients with sudden, unexplained hearing loss with or without pain

Primary Otalgia

Acute bacterial otitis externa (AOE) is an infection of the skin that lines the ear canal. Also known as swimmers ear, it is primarily caused by a bacterial infection with the primary pathogens being *Staphylococcus aureus*, *Staphylococcus epidermidis*, and *Pseudomonas*. Typically, AOE develops when there is a breach of the skin/cerumen protective barrier of the ear canal. Swimming may cause maceration of the barrier, trauma from cleaning or scratching can damage the barrier, and any external agents such as ear phones or hearing aids can disrupt the natural protective layers. Once the skin and cerumen barrier are broken, edema and inflammation ensue, leading to obstruction and increased pH in the ear canal, creating a warm environment for bacterial proliferation. Common symptoms are pain, decreased hearing, and itching. On examination, the external canal is usually erythematous and edematous with edema that may be so severe that the view of the TM is obscured; discharge may also be present (Neilan & Roland, 2010) (see Figure 2.1). Classic pain is noted when the external pinnae is pulled and on palpation of the tragus. When the TM is

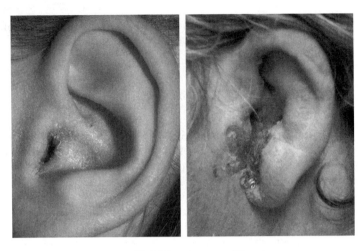

Figure 2.1 ■ Mild and severe otitis externa.
(http://ookaboo.com/o/pictures/picture/12775056/A_severe_case_of_otitis_externa)

visible, it may appear red and have signs of concomitant AOM. In the cases of OE without AOM, the TM should still be mobile with insufflation.

Treatment involves cleaning the ear canal, placing topical antibiotic/ steroid drops in contact with the skin of the ear canal, and controlling pain (Goguen, 2012). Cleaning debris from the ear canal is essential so that medication can reach the affected surface. Obvious debris (skin cells and cerumen) can be removed with suction or warm water irrigation or with a curette manually. In the cases where the TM is suspected to be ruptured or if the TM cannot be seen, patients should be referred to an ENT for thorough cleaning. Once the canal is cleared, topical agents should be used to control inflammation and infection. The typical antibiotics used are ofloxacin, ciprofloxacin, and polymyxin. Topical glucocorticoids (hydrocortisone or dexamethasone) and acidifying solutions (acetic acid or boric acid) are also helpful in decreasing inflammation and inhibiting bacterial growth. Agents such as Cipro HC and Cortisporin are good solutions that improve patient adherence (see Table 2.1 for common products used in OE treatment). If the ear canal is so edematous that getting drops into the canal is impeded, a wick should be inserted for 3 to 4 days and then reevaluated (Neilan & Roland, 2010). When a wick cannot be safely or adequately placed, the patient should be referred to an ENT for follow-up. Patients should also have oral nonsteroidal anti-inflammatory drugs (NSAIDs) for pain control. Generally, OE should improve within a week. If symptoms persist beyond 2 to 3 days, a referral to an ENT should be made. Failure to improve suggests an alternate diagnosis including contact dermatitis, carcinoma, or psoriasis (Goguen, 2011) and is best investigated by an ENT specialist.

A relatively rare complication of OE is a condition called necrotizing OE or malignant external otitis. This is a serious infection, generally seen in

Table 2.1 ■ Treatment of Otitis Externa

DISEASE CLASSIFICATION	FINDING	TREATMENT
Mild	Minor discomfort or pruritus Minimal inflammation or edema of the canal	Nonantibiotic acidifying agents with a glucocorticoid
Moderate	Intermediate pain and pruritus Partially occluded canal	Cipro HC or Cortisporin
Severe	Intense pain with a completely occluded canal May be associated with fever or periauricular erythema	Wick placement with combination therapy under the guidance of ENT Oral antibiotics when severe

Source: Goguen (2012).

immunocompromised individuals such as diabetics, resulting in osteomyelitis of the skull base. Red flags include OE that does not respond to treatment, continued discharge, pain, granulation tissue on the floor of the canal, and/or facial paralysis. These patients will usually appear ill and may have fever and will have tenderness and severe pain out of proportion to the examination. This is a life-threatening condition calling for prompt referral to an ENT specialist (Jacobsen & Antonelli, 2010).

Acute Otitis Media

AOM is inflammation of the middle ear, usually secondary to infection. AOM occurs in all age groups, but it is much more common in children and more common in boys than in girls. Lack of breastfeeding, daycare attendance, and exposure to smoke are a few of the many factors that increase the probability of developing AOM. The classic case generally follows or occurs in conjunction with URI symptoms such as cough or runny nose; the eustachian tube then fails to clear, setting up a static medium for bacterial proliferation. The predominant organisms involved are *Streptococcus pneumonia*, *Moraxella catarrhalis*, and *Haemophilus influenza*, or viruses including rhinovirus and respiratory syncytial virus (RSV). Patients will typically present with ear pain and a feeling of fullness or decreased hearing. They may have fever, irritability, vomiting, or diarrhea. Typical otoscopic examination will reveal an erythematous, bulging TM with a purulent effusion and decreased TM mobility (Ramakrishnan, Sparks, & Berryhill, 2007). On close inspection, the TM may show an air fluid level that usually represents a buildup of fluid behind the TM in the inner ear with a cloudy or opaque appearance and decreased tympanic membrane mobility (see Figures 2.2 and 2.3). The TM is often deep red or has a focal area of injection. The hallmark of AOM is a bulging TM. The external ear should be normal with no pain with manipulation of the auricle or tragus.

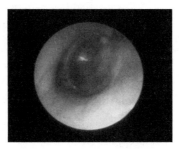

Figure 2.2 ■ Otitis media with mild erythema and fluid collection.
(© SIU BioMed/Custom Medical Stock Photo)

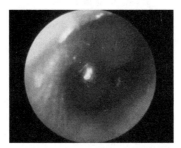

Figure 2.3 ■ Otitis media with significant erythema and fluid collection.
(© Wellcome Image Library/Custom Medical Stock Photo)

Treatment involves one of two pathways: antibiotics or a wait-and-watch approach. All patients should receive pain control.

- *Antibiotics*: In general, all patients with moderate or severe AOM, a presenting symptom of severe ear pain, or bilateral ear infections should be treated with antibiotics. Key bacteria to target include *H. influenzae, M. catarrhalis*, and *S. pneumonia*. Usual first-line drugs include amoxicillin in mild to moderate cases and Augmentin in more severe cases or in patients with systemic illness. For pediatric patients, the higher dose of 80 mg/kg twice a day should be used to ensure higher concentrations in the middle ear. Treatment duration should be 5 to 10 days. In patients with non-type-I allergies, cefdinir, cefpodoxime, or cefuroxime provide adequate coverage. Severe penicillin allergies should be provided with a macrolide such as azithromycin or clarithromycin. Patients who do not respond to Augmentin or who have more than four episodes per year should be referred to their primary care provider (PCP) or an ENT physician.
- *Wait-and-watch*: Children older than 2 years with unilateral mild disease may benefit from waiting and watching to avoid unnecessary antibiotic use. In general, mild disease is classified as minimal to no ear pain and fever less than 39°C. This approach should occur only if follow-up can be guaranteed and the parents of the patient demonstrate a clear understanding of

when to return to the clinic or when to start antibiotics. Some clinics advocate providing a prescription with instructions to fill only if the child fails to improve within 48 to 72 hours. In a CCC, it is prudent to establish a clinical policy concerning a wait-and-watch approach.

- *Pain control*: Most patients with AOM should be treated with oral NSAIDs (ibuprofen or acetaminophen). Topical drops (antipyrine, benzocaine, and glycerin) can also help alleviate pain associated with AOM and a nonperforated TM.

Follow-Up

In general, follow-up should occur within 1 to 3 days. Patients with severe pain, hearing loss, rupture of TM, loss of balance, or symptoms suggestive of infectious complications (e.g., meningitis, epidural abscess, or mastoiditis) will require urgent referral. In addition, patients who fail to improve after 3 to 5 days or those with worsening pain may benefit from an ENT referral.

Otitis Media With Effusion

As opposed to AOM, OME is a noninfectious process that causes feelings of ear fullness and decreased hearing as a result of fluid buildup in the middle ear. This is most typically caused by allergies but can also accompany a viral URI. On inspection, the TM is usually immobile and may be retracted; however, it is usually normal in color and should not appear red. Treatment involves reversing eustachian tube dysfunction (ETD) or treating the underlying process of allergies or URI. This condition will usually resolve spontaneously; however, when it does not, an ENT referral is warranted.

Eustachian Tube Dysfunction

The eustachian tube "vents" the middle ear by periodically opening and equalizing pressure. When this tube fails to vent, fluid and pressure can build up in the middle ear. ETD can occur secondary to any type of inflammation (infection, allergies, and pollutants) or from various secondary causes such as trauma, reflux, or even hormonal changes. Patients will present with ear pain, ear fullness or ear plugging, hearing loss, or tinnitus. A popping or crackling sound in the ear is not uncommon. Patients may also report that they feel like they are speaking in an echo chamber or container causing them to hear their own voice. On examination, the middle ear usually appears normal, but an effusion may be present. Insufflation is an important part of the examination, because the TM will often appear normal but be immobile. ETD often leads to AOM and hence should be treated when possible. In general, treatment of the underlying etiology will treat ETD. Treatment of sinusitis, allergic rhinitis, or reflux with decongestants (pseudoephedrine or phenylephrine) and antibiotics when warranted can alleviate ETD.

Bullous Myringitis

Bullous myringitis is an acute bacterial infection resulting in large blebs or bullae on the TM and can be extremely painful (McCormick et al., 2003). Like AOM, it is more prevalent in children. Additionally, the causative organisms are similar, and this should guide treatment (Neilan & Roland, 2010). It will be important to inform patients that they may experience drainage if the bullae rupture but that this is no cause for alarm. Treatment includes pain control and antibiotics when a bacterial source is considered.

Traumatic TM Rupture

The TM can also rupture because of penetrating trauma (e.g., Q-tip), blunt trauma (a punch or slap to the side of the head), or with barotrauma. Barotrauma is a phenomenon in which pressure in the middle ear space decreases rapidly, and fluid and blood are drawn in from the surrounding tissues; the sudden change in pressure may be very uncomfortable; it is most often associated with activities such as flying and scuba diving. The TM typically appears bruised or blue because of bleeding, and if the change in pressure is severe enough, the TM may rupture (Neilan & Roland, 2010).

Ruptured TM typically resolves with time; however, it may take several weeks for hearing to return to normal and for the TM to heal. Analgesics may be necessary, along with decongestants or nasal steroid sprays to aid proper eustachian tube function. Patients with persistent effusion may need to refer an ENT specialist for myringotomy and drainage (Mirza & Richardson, 2005).

Cerumen and Cerumen Impaction

Cerumen is a protective coating that naturally develops in the ear canal to protect the lining of the canal from trauma or infection. Occasionally, cerumen can build up to the point that the TM cannot be seen. Rarely, cerumen impaction itself can cause symptoms of ear fullness or decreased hearing or cause pain or tenderness. Accumulation can also cause dizziness or tinnitus, although these, too, are rare. As cerumen accumulates, it can harden into a dense concretion ranging in color from white to dark red.

Removal: Cerumen should be removed when a patient presents with ear complaints and the TM cannot be easily seen; the symptoms may also be secondary to the impaction. Asymptomatic cerumen impaction found during an examination of a patient with non-ENT-related complaint does not require removal.

Removal techniques: There are various techniques for cerumen removal; success is dependent on provider skill or comfort with the various techniques. Providers in the CCC should become familiar with all of the following:

1. Cerumenolytics: Using drops to break up cerumen is a useful first-line approach to patients with impaction. Drops should not be used if there

is suspicion of TM rupture as indicated by ear pain or drainage. Patients should use Debrox® drops, over-the-counter (OTC) hydrogen peroxide, or mineral oil for 3 to 5 days and should return to the clinic for visual inspection and manual removal, or irrigation if removal was incomplete.

2. Manual removal: Under direct visualization using a hook, a curette, or forceps, cerumen can safely be removed. Manual removal is the safest form when the TM cannot be seen and there is suspicion of TM damage.

3. Irrigation: Using warm water with or without a bacteriostatic agent, the ear canal can be irrigated to physically flush out cerumen. There are various tools including jet-powered canal irrigators and simple irrigation tips that can be placed on a syringe to avoid direct pressure on the TM. In the cases of hardened cerumen, a cerumenolytic agent should be used for a few days before irrigation.

Complications can develop including dizziness (due to cold water in the inner ear), trauma to the canal (manual manipulation), and allergic reactions (to cerumenolytics).

COMPLICATIONS OF PRIMARY EAR INFECTIONS

Mastoiditis

Mastoiditis is an infection of the mastoid air spaces that are connected to the middle ear; it is an uncommon complication of AOM in the United States. Patients will present with pain and fever and will often appear toxic. They have pain when the mastoid bone is palpated. Patients who have persistent pain despite appropriate and adequate treatment with antibiotic therapy should be referred to an ENT for evaluation (Ramakrishnan et al., 2007).

Spontaneous Rupture of the Tympanic Membrane

Another complication of AOM can be rupture of the TM, which occurs when the pressure of the middle ear increases, causing an outward bowing against the TM and eventual rupture. The patient will typically present with ear discharge that developed after severe, increasing ear pain followed by a sudden cessation of pain and decrease in hearing. These patients should be treated with oral and topical antibiotics such as ofloxacin otic. Most tears will heal; however, patients should follow up with an ENT for hearing testing and confirmation of healing.

Foreign Bodies

FBs in the ear can cause varying levels of discomfort depending on their size and can also be very distressing to parents. Commonly found objects include beads, bugs, pebbles, hearing-aid batteries, and cotton-swab tips, to name a few—treatment is primarily removal. Most objects do not require immediate removal, with the exception of hearing-aid batteries, which may cause alkali burns (Ely et al., 2008). Small, nonembedded objects (e.g., bugs, kernels of corn, beads) can be easily flushed out. Items that are wedged in the canal or items that could swell in size with irrigation (e.g., cotton, sponges, beans, facial tissue) should be removed with instrumentation. Items that are embedded into the canal or TM are best referred to an ENT. Hearing-aid batteries that are not easily removed with instrumentation should also be referred.

The key to removing FBs is often hands-free lighting. If your clinic does not have a light source, a camping headlight is an inexpensive item that may come in handy. If after the object is removed, the canal is abraded or scratched, antibiotic drops should be considered to prevent infection.

Removing FBs in children poses a special challenge, requiring particular consideration of immobilization for safe removal. If the FB cannot be safely removed, referral to an ENT is recommended.

Ramsay Hunt Syndrome (Herpes Zoster Oticus)

Patients with Ramsay Hunt syndrome will typically present with ear pain; a red, swollen external ear with vesicular rash; and facial paralysis. Other presenting complaints may include hearing loss, tinnitus, and vertigo (Ely et al., 2008). This disease represents a reactivation of the chicken pox virus in the distribution of nerves that serve the outer ear. Treatment should include the same antiviral therapy and pain control that would be prescribed for any typical zoster infection. Patients should then be followed for pain control, secondary infection, and resolution. If hearing loss is present, referral to an ENT is indicated.

Cellulitis/Chondritis

Inflammation of the skin and cartilage of the external ear may produce pain, redness, or swelling. Cellulitis/chondritis can develop with OE or with trauma that breaks the skin, such as an abrasion, insect bite, or piercing, and causes an infection. *Pseudomonas* and *S. aureus* are typical pathogens. Treatment requires oral and topical antibiotics. Fluoroquinolones are a good choice, because they cover both gram-positive and gram-negative organisms (Neilan & Roland, 2010). There is a high risk of cosmetic deformity with these types of infections; thus, if an abscess is suspected, referral should be made for incision and drainage (I&D).

Secondary Otalgia

Dental Disease

Otalgia from dental disease may include caries, dental abscess, impacted wisdom teeth, or pulpitis. When the ear examination is normal, providers should do a very careful oral examination, because dental disease is a likely source (Ely et al., 2008). Referral to an appropriate dental care provider is indicated if abnormalities are found. It is also important to keep in mind that treating patients for dental issues in the convenient care environment is not advised within the constraints of the clinical setting.

Temporomandibular Joint Dysfunction

TMJ dysfunction is characterized by pain and/or crepitus in the TM joint with opening and closing of the mouth. Patients may experience pain and popping or shifting of the joint with chewing. Palpation of the TM joint should be done when the otic examination is normal. Patients will typically complain of tenderness on palpation, and crepitus or shifting may or may not be appreciated. Treatment includes having the patient follow a soft diet, take anti-inflammatories, avoid chewing gum, and apply heat (Neilan & Roland, 2010). The patient should also be referred to a dentist because other treatment options such as oral splints and bite correction may be indicated.

Pharyngitis

Pharyngitis, tonsillitis, or lesions of the pharynx can cause referred pain to the ear. Patients will typically but not always complain of a sore throat as well (Neilan & Roland, 2010). Again, it is very important to examine the oral cavity following a normal otic examination. A single aphthous ulcer on the tonsil or edge of the soft palate can cause pain that is referred into the ear, especially with swallowing. Treatment is dependent on causation.

Temporal Arteritis

Temporal pain and tenderness make up the classic presentation for temporal arteritis in adults; however, the discomfort can also involve the ear. Other presenting symptoms may include headache, malaise, fever, decreased appetite, and weight loss. Many patients may not have temporal area tenderness; however, a large percentage of patients will have one of the following: tenderness, decreased or absent pulse, or prominence or beading of the artery (Smetana & Shmerling, 2002). It can be beneficial to have the patient locate the pain by pointing to the area of concern. It is extremely important to recognize temporal arteritis, because it can lead to permanent blindness; if it is suspected, advise the patient for an urgent appointment with his or her PCP or to an emergency room. Have a high suspicion for this disorder in elderly patients presenting with headache, vision complaints, and tenderness to palpation of the temporal area of their forehead.

Tumors of the Head and Neck

In the case of head and neck tumors, otalgia may be the initial or only presenting symptom. Unexplained, persistent otalgia in an adult requires a thorough evaluation of the nasopharynx, oropharynx, and larynx to rule out an occult process. Neoplastic disease should also be considered, particularly if the pain is accompanied by weight loss, odynophagia, dysphagia, or change in vocal quality. Risk factors include age (>50), tobacco use (smokeless included), and excessive alcohol intake. These patients are best referred to an ENT for a full evaluation (Neilan & Roland, 2010).

Parotitis

The parotid glands are located anterior and inferior to the ear, and their infection or inflammation can cause referred ear pain. Parotitis is usually easily diagnosed by an astute clinician, who will detect tenderness or swelling of these glands. Treatment of the problem (obstruction) or infection with antibiotics will alleviate these symptoms.

Case Resolution: Based on the symptoms and the patient's self-report, the diagnosis appears to be barotrauma causing TM rupture. Because of the size of the rupture and the mechanism behind this patient's TM perforation, referral to an ENT was indicated. With the patient's hearing being decreased, and history of trauma, an audiogram is indicated to evaluate the degree of hearing loss and to rule out an ossicular chain injury. The patient was started on an antibiotic drop with middle-ear indication because of the exposure to dirty water.

When perforations are greater than 5% to 10%, it is unlikely that the TM will spontaneously heal. Surgical correction is not crucial, but patients with chronic perforations may have hearing loss and remain open to infection.

SUMMARY

Ear pain is one of the most common complaints seen in any medical care setting for both pediatric and adult patients. There is a wide range of complexity and origin for the complaint, and it is extremely important for providers to be aware of primary and secondary causes of otalgia, along with the common presenting symptoms, to help guide management.

3

Red Eye and Other Eye Complaints

TRACEY J. KNIESS AND SANDRA F. RYAN

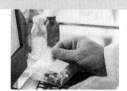

APPROACH TO COMMON EYE COMPLAINTS IN THE CONVENIENT CARE SETTING

Red eye and other eye complaints are commonly seen in primary care (Cronau, Kankanala, & Mauger, 2010) and account for 1% to 2% of all ambulatory office visits (Wu, 2012). Infectious conjunctivitis is the most common presenting eye-related complaint seen in the convenient care clinic. Most eye complaints are easily managed in the convenient care setting; however, vigilance must be maintained to identify vision-threatening or more serious conditions that require referral to ophthalmology.

Case Study: A 12-year-old boy is brought to the clinic by his mother, complaining of red eyes for 3 days. The mother states that the redness started in the right eye 3 days ago, and today, it has spread to the left eye. The child denies pain or photophobia but states his eyes are "crusted shut" in the morning. He also denies any trauma or foreign body sensation, or pain but complains of a watery to mucus-like discharge from both eyes. He has no known drug allergies (NKDA) and does not wear contact lenses. On review of symptoms (ROS), he denies recent cough, cold, or other illness, trauma, any vision changes, ear or throat pain, and arthralgia or myalgia.

HISTORY AND REVIEW OF SYSTEMS

Patient history is crucial to accurate diagnosis of red eye. The history should clearly document the duration of symptoms, bilateral or unilateral eye involvement, drainage (watery vs. purulent, continuous or worse in the morning), contact lens use, pain, photophobia, allergy history, and systemic illnesses. It is also important to ask and document whether vision is affected. Patients should be questioned about foreign-body sensation, which requires distinguishing between a subjective sensation of a foreign body (e.g., eyes feel gritty or as though there is sand in them) and an objective sensation (patient is visibly in pain and has a hard time opening the eye). In general, subjective sensations may be conjunctivitis. Objective symptoms of a foreign body, however, generally indicate damage to the cornea and often require referral. It is also important to question about known injury or trauma, whether any of the patient's contacts have similar symptoms and have any treatments been tried at home (Tarabishy & Jeng, 2008). In addition, it is also important to elicit any history of eye surgery.

Fluorescein Staining

Staining of the cornea is a technique used to identify abrasions, lacerations, or foreign bodies on the cornea. This technique is useful in the examination of a red eye that is associated with trauma or a subjective sensation of a foreign body.

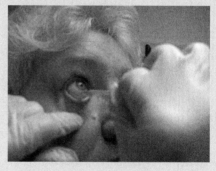

To perform the examination, confirm that there is no open globe (irregular pupil), blunt trauma, or penetrating trauma. First, instill 1 or 2 drops of a rapid, short-duration topical ophthalmologic anesthesia (Uphold & Graham, 2003a) and instill the fluorescein stain into the lower lid. The strip should be moistened with saline, which allows the fluorescein to drain into the inferior cul-de-sac of the eye. The patient should then blink to evenly distribute the stain. Fluorescein stains the basement membrane, which is only exposed when the epithelial layer is impaired.

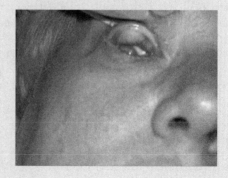

Reexamine the eye using a cobalt blue light or a Wood's lamp that will fluoresce any corneal abrasions. The upper lid should then be everted to examine the upper tarsal conjunctiva and remove any foreign body. This is done by having the patient look downward; grasp the eye lashes of the upper lid and raise it upward while applying gentle pressure on the tarsal plate with a cotton swab (Uphold & Graham, 2003).

Remove any foreign body with saline flush or by sweeping a moistened cotton swab across the conjunctival area. The lid will return to normal anatomical position when the cotton swab is removed from the tarsal plate and the patient blinks several times. Have the patient look upward, gently pull the lower lid downward, and examine the inferior cul-de-sac for foreign body (Uphold & Graham, 2003). If there is severe pain or difficulty removing any foreign body, the patient should be referred to an ophthalmologist. After the examination is complete, flush the eye with normal saline to remove any excess dye.

PHYSICAL EXAMINATION

Physical examination of the patient with a red eye must include blood pressure, visual inspection of the eyelids and lachrymal sac, visual acuity, pupil size, shape, reaction to light, conjunctival injection, and preauricular adenopathy (Tarabishy & Jeng, 2008). A corrected Snellen visual acuity test should be performed on each eye individually (Shah, 2011). Failure to document visual acuity presents a significant medico-legal risk. If the patient wears corrective lenses but does not have them available, visual acuity should be measured through a pin hole (Shah, 2011). When performing the penlight examination, comment on the reaction to light and the size of the pupil. Note any lid swelling or asymmetry, discharge (quality and quantity), obvious foreign body, abrasion, or hyphema (Uphold & Graham, 2003b). In addition, look for any injection of the conjunctiva. The pattern of redness can be diagnostic; when the redness is spread throughout the bulbar and palpebral conjunctiva, it is more consistent with a primary conjunctivitis. When the redness is centered around the limbus and then diminishes (ciliary flush), one needs to be more concerned about conditions such as iritis or acute glaucoma. Extraocular muscles should also be tested, and comment on the skin surrounding the eyes as well.

Red Flags

If any of the following turn up during the history or the physical examination, referral elsewhere may be required:

- Postoperative pain or redness
- Pain or photophobia severe enough to prevent examination

- History of blast, blunt, or sharp trauma
- Herpetic lesions or dendritic pattern on cornea
- Retained foreign body
- Corneal rust ring
- Contact lens wearers (in certain cases)
- Limbal flush/uveitis
- Loss of visual acuity: In general, loss of vision or vision reduction in the setting of a red eye is a harbinger of a more worrisome diagnosis.
- Hyphema: A meniscus of blood in the bottom part of the pupil; this condition suggests bleeding into the anterior eye and requires a referral.
- Hypopyon: This is a layer of white blood cells that can be seen on visual inspection in the anterior chamber of the eye. This requires emergent referral to an ophthalmologist.
- Fixed pupil suggestive of acute glaucoma

Continuation of Case Study: On physical examination, he appeared to be a well-developed 12-year-old boy. His temperature was 37 Celsius, with a pulse of 78, respirations of 12, and blood pressure of 102/62. His lungs were clear, and he was without rhinorrhea with clear TM. His visual acuity was at 20/20 in each eye without correction.

Pupils are round and reactive to light and accommodation, conjunctival injection in both eyes, no chemosis or limbal flush, globe intact, mucoid exudate noted bilaterally on upper eyelashes. When the discharge is wiped away, watery discharge reaccumulates. No ptosis, no erythema of lids. One cm preauricular node enlargement right only. Tetracaine ophthalmic solution two drops instilled in each eye and fluorescein dye instilled. No areas of increased uptake or foreign body noted in either eye. Excess fluorescein stain removed with gentle saline flush.

RED EYE SYMPTOMS USUALLY TREATED IN THE CONVENIENT CARE SETTING

Conjunctivitis

Acute conjunctivitis is described by Wu (2012) as inflammation of the mucous membrane that lines the inner surface of the eye lids and the outer surface of the globe of the eye (the conjunctiva). The etiology includes bacterial and viral infections, allergic response, and nonspecific irritant induced by or secondary to a systemic disease process (Wu, 2012). It usually presents as unilateral or bilateral red and itchy eye.

Viral Conjunctivitis

The most common cause of conjunctivitis is a viral etiology (Sethuraman & Kamat, 2009) (see Figure 3.1). These infections are often self-limiting and may take several weeks to resolve. Viral conjunctivitis is typically caused by

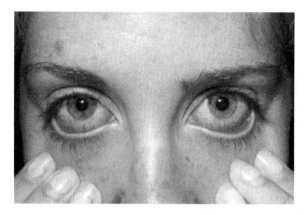

Figure 3.1 ■ Viral conjunctivitis with uniform irritation and inflammation. Although the discharge is classically watery, patients may report waking up with matted eyelids. A sandy foreign-body sensation is common.
(© Custom Medical Stock Photo)

adenovirus (most common) or Coxsackie virus, enterovirus, varicella, measles, mumps, or influenza (Wu, 2012). It is often associated with an upper respiratory infection and will present with other respiratory tract symptoms. The case may be unilateral, but within 24 hours, most become bilateral. Patients will often complain of pus when they wake up in the morning with matted eyelids. On closer inspection, it is evident that the discharge during the day is watery but accumulates at night, appearing matted in the morning. When the matted discharge is cleared from the corner of the eye, it usually reaccumulates as a watery discharge. The patient will often describe a gritty sensation.

Preauricular nodes may be tender. Patients may complain of a foreign body sensation but should be able to open their eye for examination with limited pain. The injection will be fairly uniform throughout the entire conjunctiva, and there may be a follicular reaction of the inferior tarsal conjunctiva that will present as small whitish round plaques on the conjunctiva. The patient should not have pain or true photophobia, and vision should not be impaired.

Nonherpetic viral conjunctivitis is treated symptomatically with cold compresses, artificial tears, and topical antihistamine/decongestants (e.g., Naphcon-A). However, although this is not a recommended practice, antibiotic ophthalmic treatment may be required before the patient is permitted to return to work or school or if a distinction between bacterial or viral etiology cannot be made. An over-the-counter, Clinical Laboratory Improvement Act–waived test is available to test for adenovirus, and positive results can avoid unnecessary antibiotic use. Patients should follow up with an ophthalmologist in 5 to 7 days if symptoms do not improve, or sooner if symptoms worsen (Wu, 2012). Patients should stay absent from school or work until discharge stops or until 24 hours after the initiation of antibiotics if they were warranted.

Bacterial Conjunctivitis

According to the Centers for Disease Control and Prevention (CDC, 2012), the most common bacteria causing conjunctivitis in the United States are *Staphylococcus aureus, Haemophilus* species (children), and *Streptococcus pneumoniae*. Bacterial conjunctivitis is more common in children than in adults. It is highly contagious and spreads most often through direct hand to eye contact (Cronau et al., 2010). Bacterial conjunctivitis has a more rapid onset than viral conjunctivitis and produces a discharge that is thicker in consistency and tends to persist throughout the day (see Figure 3.2). It usually starts in one eye, but because of its highly contagious nature, it often spreads to the second eye within 48 hours. In general, bacterial conjunctivitis should not have photophobia or visual impairment when purulent material is removed.

Bacterial and viral conjunctivitis are difficult to distinguish. One distinguishing feature is that during the day viral conjunctivitis tends to be mild but during the night causes a crusting that generates matted eyes in the morning. Bacterial conjunctivitis, on the contrary, has a thicker discharge that persists through the day. A good clinical test is to wipe away the discharge in the clinic with a piece of gauze. Purulent discharge that accumulates within a minute or two typically indicates a bacterial infection, whereas a more watery discharge is consistent with a viral infection. In addition, the redness in a bacterial infection tends to be more pronounced at the fornices (Mahmood & Narang, 2008).

Treatment for non–sexually transmitted disease (STD) bacterial conjunctivitis with no comorbidity is broad-spectrum topical antibiotics such as bacitracin/polymyxin B or erythromycin ophthalmic ointment. Ointments require less frequent application and cause vision impairment; they are best used in pediatric patients. Drops are easier to apply and are more appropriate for adult patients. Bacterial conjunctivitis is generally benign and should improve within 2 to 4 days of starting treatment. Failure to improve within 4 days requires referral for cultures and further investigation. One exception to this is in sexually active patients who present with extremely copious discharge

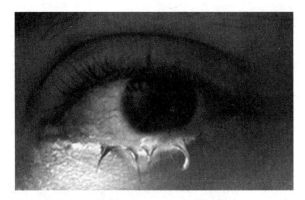

Figure 3.2 ■ Bacterial conjunctivitis can be distinguished from viral causes when a thicker discharge is present, which redevelops immediately after being wiped away.
(http://ookaboo.com/o/pictures/picture/23887100/Eye_with_conjunctivitis_exuding_pus)

(aka hyperacute conjunctivitis) and a tender, red eye. With these symptoms, be suspicious for *Neisseria gonorrhoeea*, which requires urgent, same-day referral. In addition to excessive amounts of discharge, patients will have lid swelling and redness and preauricular lymphadenopathy.

Patients with dry eye, immunosuppression, or diabetes mellitus are treated with cefazolin plus gentamicin or tobramycin ophthalmic every 15 to 60 minutes around the clock with follow-up the next day with ophthalmology. Contact lens wearers need to be treated for *Pseudomonas aeruginosa* with tobramycin or ciprofloxacin ophthalmic drops, also 1 drop every 15 to 60 minutes around the clock and also with follow-up with ophthalmology the next day for taper instructions (Sanford Guide, 2012). Patient education includes good hand-washing instructions, avoiding sharing towels, and disposing of eye makeup and contact lenses. Antibiotic resistance to ocular isolates is also increasing (Haas, Pillar, Torres, Morris, & Sahm, 2011). Results from the Antibiotic Resistance Monitoring in Ocular Microorganisms (ARMOR) study reveal resistance to one or more antibiotics among ocular bacterial pathogens. As with prescribing any antibiotic, resistance trends should be considered before initiating empiric treatment of common eye infections.

Allergic Conjunctivitis

Allergic conjunctivitis represents an immune response to foreign allergens. It may be an acute allergic reaction to an antigen (e.g., cat dander) or may be seasonal allergy related (e.g., pollen). It will present as itchy eyes with watery discharge, burning, photophobia, and occasionally conjunctival edema. The diagnosis is usually made clinically and can often be confused with infectious conjunctivitis; however, the presence of itch often suggests an allergic component. On examination, the patient will have a global injection of the conjunctiva affecting both the eyes. There may be associated eye swelling, and when discharge is present, it will be watery.

Treatment is predominantly symptomatic, with instructions for good eye hygiene (do not rub eyes; use artificial tears [they dilute the allergen]). Topical antihistamines are helpful during acute flares and can be used up to four times a day but should be used for no more than 2 weeks at a time (Naphcon-A, Visine-A, and Opcon-A). In addition to allergen avoidance, cool compresses can also relieve symptoms. For patients with frequent episodes, a topical antihistamine and mast cell stabilizer (olopatadine, azelastine, and ketotifen) is useful to help diminish or prevent frequency of attacks. Oral antihistamines such as loratadine, fexofenadine, or cetirizine also play a role for frequent or more irritating symptoms. Patients who do not improve after 2 to 3 weeks of treatment should be referred to an ophthalmologist.

Subconjunctival Hemorrhage

Presents as a distinctly red area of extravasated blood beneath the surface of the eye (see Figure 3.3). While visually very concerning, this is a benign condition that is usually asymptomatic. The patient should not have any foreign

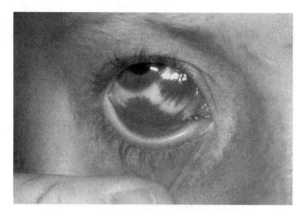

Figure 3.3 ■ A subconjunctival hemorrhage, although concerning to the patient, these benign small bleeds self-resolve in 2 to 4 weeks.
(© Biomedical Communications/Medical Stock Photo)

body sensation or visual acuity problems. This diagnosis can be a sign of uncontrolled hypertension; hence, it is important to check blood pressure. No treatment is needed, and the blood will slowly reabsorb over a course of a few weeks. Patients on anticoagulants should be referred for anticoagulant level checks when appropriate.

Corneal Abrasions

Corneal abrasions are scratches of the epithelium, which covers the cornea, most commonly due to trauma or damage from a foreign body, including contact lenses. Patients will present with a chief complaint of eye pain and will have some degree of distress when opening the eye. The pain can be severe and is often associated with photophobia.

It is important to distinguish between a corneal abrasion secondary to trauma and an epithelium defect due to an infectious process. The two can be distinguished based on a history suggestive of trauma or on physical examination. On inspection of the eye, look for signs of obvious trauma. An irregular or fixed pupil, orbital deformity, hyphema, or hypopyon mandate same-day referral. It is occasionally necessary to use a topical anesthetic to allow for inspection. Corneal abrasions may be detectable with a penlight examination when large and with fluorescein staining when small. Patterns of dendritic branching may be concerning for herpetic lesions. If an abrasion is detected, treatment consists of topical antibiotics to prevent superinfection. Good choices include erythromycin ointment, Polytrim, ciprofloxacin, or ofloxacin. Pain control should also be addressed with oral pain medication and topical cycloplegics (homatropine and cyclopentolate). Patients with cornea abrasions should have follow-up scheduled within a few days or within

24 to 48 hours if symptoms are not relieved. Suspected corneal abrasions in contact lens wearers should be referred to an ophthalmologist.

CONDITIONS REQUIRING URGENT REFERRAL

A number of conditions are serious enough to typically warrant referral to an emergency room or other form of urgent care.

Trauma

If an open globe is suspected, a hard shield should be placed over the injured eye, and the patient should be immediately transported to an ophthalmologist or an emergency department (Uphold & Graham, 2003). If there are no hard eye shields available, the lid from a sterile urine cup may be used.

Foreign Bodies

If patient history suggests that the foreign body of the conjunctiva is sand or dirt or is related to contact lens use, the eye must be examined for trapped debris under the upper lid or cornea. Any retained foreign body of the upper lid or cornea may require referral if it is not easily removed. Metal foreign bodies embedded on the cornea will form a rust ring within a few hours. Rust rings should most likely be removed by an ophthalmologist.

Bacterial Keratitis

Keratitis is inflammation of the cornea (as opposed to the conjunctiva in conjunctivitis). Patients with keratitis will have a red eye and objective signs of a foreign body sensation. They will typically have a hard time opening their eye because of pain. Patients who wear contact lenses are at higher risk of developing keratitis, as are immunosuppressed patients. The main difference between this and bacterial conjunctivitis is damage to and infection of the cornea, which can be seen as corneal opacity or a white spot. This lesion can usually be seen with a penlight and will be detected with fluorescein staining. In severe cases, patients may have a hypopyon, and most will have purulent discharge. Presentation of a red eye with photophobia and objective signs of a foreign body should have a high suspicion for keratitis and should be referred the same day to an ophthalmologist.

Special Cases: Contact Lens Wearers

Contact lens use predisposes wearers to more serious complications of eye infections and eye complaints. Heightened awareness is required, along with a lower threshold for referral to ophthalmology. Some common diagnoses in contact lens wearers include the following:

Corneal Epithelial Defects: Trauma, oxygen debt, chemical toxicity, or drying can cause the epithelium behind the lens to become compromised, which will present as tearing, photophobia, pain, and decreased vision. On physical examination, there will be scattered fluorescein uptake. Contacts should not be worn, and the patient should be seen by an ophthalmologist. It is usually self-limiting.

Mechanical Corneal Abrasion: Poor-fitting contacts, contact defects, or trauma when inserting or removing contacts can cause a very painful eye. Contact lens wearers with corneal abrasions are at increased risk for bacterial ulcerative keratitis. To protect against possible *Pseudomonas* superinfection, prophylactic topical antibiotics such as ciprofloxacin or ofloxacin should be used. Patients should be referred to an ophthalmologist the next day and contact use discontinued.

Contact Lens–Related Infectious Keratitis: Patients will present with a red, painful eye. They often have photophobia and may have diminished visual acuity. Contact lenses should be removed for the examination. Fluorescein staining will reveal a corneal epithelial defect, and hypopyon will develop in severe cases. If infectious keratitis is suspected, patients should be referred to an ophthalmologist.

Conjunctivitis: Patients presenting with conjunctivitis who wear contact lenses need to be covered for *Pseudomonas*. If symptoms do not improve within 24 hours, patients should be referred to an ophthalmologist.

Herpes Simplex Infection

When herpes simplex virus causes conjunctivitis, it can lead to corneal damage. Patients with herpes conjunctivitis will present with a red eye, watery discharge, and a foreign body sensation. The pain and subjective burning sensation help distinguish it from adenovirus conjunctivitis. These patients should undergo fluorescein staining to rule out a corneal ulcer. If the virus is causing just conjunctivitis and there is no corneal lesion, treatment is topical antiviral medication such as trifluridine 1% or vidarabine 3% ointment.

If the patient presents with photophobia or has a lesion, more aggressive treatment is required, because herpetic lesions on the cornea can produce scarring and can cause lasting visual changes—hence, urgent referral is needed. Herpetic keratitis is diagnosed when a classic dendritic-patterned ulcer of the cornea is seen on penlight examination or with fluorescein staining. According to the *2012 Sanford Guide to Antimicrobial Therapy*, herpetic conjunctivitis is treated with trifluridine 1% drops, one drop every

2 hours up to nine drops a day and famciclovir 500mg every 8 hours for 10 days or oral acyclovir. During the consultation, recommend that patient follow up with an ophthalmologist, typically within 1 to 2 days; same-day referral can also be prudent. When herpetic infections are suspected, steroid eye drops should be avoided.

Iritis

Inflammation of the anterior uveal tract. Patients usually present with a red eye that is centrally located as a red ring around the iris (ciliary flush) and with photophobia. A key to this diagnosis is pain with direct and indirect penlight (in both the affected and the unaffected eye because of the consensual response). There is usually no discharge. Iritis is best treated by an ophthalmologist.

Acute Closed-Angle Glaucoma

Acute glaucoma is one of the most emergent conditions that can cause a red eye. It develops when the peripheral iris prevents the outflow of anterior chamber fluid, resulting in a rise in intraocular pressure. Patients, most often the elderly, present with a severe headache, nausea, and even vomiting or abdominal pain. They will have a red eye with blurred vision, and they may report seeing halos around light. They are usually in obvious pain and have a dull ache in their eye. The eye will be red with ciliary flush and a pupil that may be fixed in mid-dilation. As the intraocular pressure rises, symptoms become more severe. The diagnosis is made by measuring intraocular pressure and confirmed when pressure is greater than 45 mmHg. This condition requires emergent referral, preferably by emergency medical service (EMS).

Hyphema

A collection of red blood cells in the anterior chamber of the eye usually secondary to trauma. It can cause staining of the cornea and requires emergent referral (see Figure 3.4).

Hypopyon

A collection of white blood cells in the anterior chamber of the eye secondary to an infectious process. The conjunctiva will be red with a layer of white blood cells accumulating secondary to gravity. This is an ocular emergency and will require immediate ophthalmology referral.

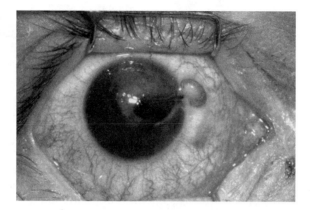

Figure 3.4 ■ Hyphema, or blood in the anterior chamber of the eye, usually follows trauma and requires an urgent ophthalmology referral.
(© Wellcome Images/Custom Medical Stock Photo)

DIFFERENTIAL DIAGNOSIS: OTHER EYE COMPLAINTS

Chalazion

Patients with chalazion may present with a complaint of eyelid swelling and a painless pea-sized nodule on their eyelid (see Figure 3.5). The lesion represents a chronic inflammatory condition that develops from an obstructed tear gland. Most often these lesions resolve on their own, but warm compresses up to five

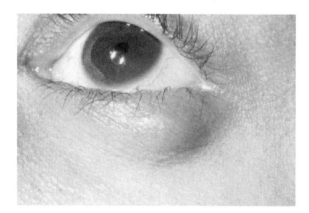

Figure 3.5 ■ Chalazion: A small nodular swelling that represents a cyst in the eyelid caused by inflammation of a blocked meibomian gland.
(© Science Photo Library/Custom Medical Stock Photo)

times a day can accelerate drainage and healing. Large lesions that obstruct vision can be incised by an ophthalmologist.

Hordeolum

Patients with hordeolum will present with an inflamed eyelid that usually has one site of swelling representing a localized infection. Most swollen lids will drain spontaneously when augmented by warm compresses up to five times a day. Swelling that does not resolve within 1 or 2 weeks or that is large enough to obstruct vision requires incision and drainage, which should be done by an ophthalmologist.

Chalazions or hordeolums that persist or that have irregular appearances or discolorations should be referred because eyelid carcinomas can be formed, including basal cell and squamous cell carcinoma.

Orbital and Preseptal Cellulitis

Conditions of orbital or preseptal cellulitis represent bacterial infections of the eyelid and surrounding skin (preseptal) or orbital structures (orbital); the hallmark difference is pain with extraocular motion in orbital cellulitis (see Figure 3.6). Both usually require imaging in the form of a computerized tomography (CT) scan of the orbits and thus are best treated in an alternate setting.

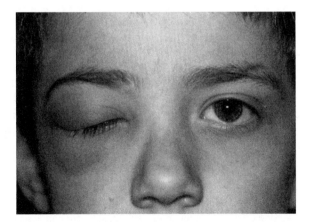

Figure 3.6 ■ Orbital cellulitis represents an infection of the eye and is hallmarked by pain with extraocular movement. It requires a CT scan for diagnosis.
(© Science Photo Library/Custom Medical Stock Photo)

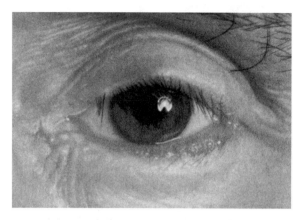

Figure 3.7 ■ Blepharitis is swelling or inflammation of the eyelids, usually where the eyelash hair follicles are located.
(© Custom Medical Stock Photo)

Blepharitis

Blepharitis is a chronic inflammation of the eyelids that presents as a crusting lesion and eye irritation (see Figure 3.7). Some patients will present with isolated crusting on their eyelids, caused by excess seborrhea production or a staph infection. In others, the inner portion of the eyelid has an over-productive meibomian gland, which can lead to itchy, red eyes with a foreign body sensation and excessive tearing. Physical examination will reveal red and swollen eyelids with flaking or scaling. Key to the diagnosis is to closely inspect the eyelids, which should be slightly inflamed and show crusting between the lashes. Because this is a chronic condition, treatment is focused on lid hygiene, which includes warm compresses applied for 10 minutes at a time four to five times a day. In addition, lids should be washed with diluted baby shampoo and lightly scrubbed to remove debris. Massage can also be used on the edge of the lid to promote gland drainage. In cases where hygiene does not solve the problem, topical antibiotics applied on the lid margin up to four times a day can be helpful; bacitracin, azithromycin, and erythromycin are all effective. Recalcitrant blepharitis should be referred to an ophthalmologist for oral antibiotics and topical steroids.

Case Resolution: Based on the symptoms of watery discharge and a tender lymph node, a diagnosis of viral conjunctivitis was made. The patient's mother was instructed on good eye hygiene including thorough hand washing, not touching his eyes, not sharing towels or washcloths, and changing pillowcases often. They were instructed to return in 3 days if not improving or sooner if symptoms change or worsen.

SUMMARY

There are numerous causes of red eye, the most common being bacterial, viral, and allergic conjunctivitis. These conditions can be easily diagnosed and treated in the convenient care clinic. A comprehensive history and physical are the keys to correct diagnosis and treatment. Any vision-threatening illnesses or eye injuries must be immediately referred for further evaluation and treatment.

4

Approach to the Patient With a Sore Throat

LYNETTE SULLIVAN AND JOSHUA RIFF

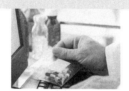

Acute pharyngitis accounts for almost 12 million ambulatory care visits in the United States and is one of the five most common primary diagnoses in a convenient care setting. Pharyngitis is characterized as an inflammatory syndrome of the pharynx and/or tonsils caused by several different groups of microorganisms (Aung, 2011). In evaluating sore throats in the convenient care setting, there are three important steps: rule out clinical emergencies; make a diagnosis—in particular, determine whether it is bacterial in nature; and relieve symptoms. Up to 70% of cases are viral in origin, and careful patient education and support are essential. Approximately 15% to 30% of all cases of pharyngitis in children and up to 30% in adults are bacterial, with the most clinically significant etiology being Group A β-hemolytic streptococcus (GABHS). It is important to understand how to diagnose GABHS in order to avoid unnecessary antibiotic use.

Case Study: A 10-year-old female presents to the clinic with a sore throat, fever, headache, stomachache, body aches, and chills. Her mother states that her daughter started to complain of headaches 3 days before and seemed "less like herself," wanting to rest on the couch and eating much less than usual. She woke up this morning with a fever of 101.9° and complained of a sore throat that was worse with swallowing, along with some nausea; she denies any vomiting, ear pain, runny nose, cough, shortness of breath, or rashes. The patient's mother does say that her daughter's voice sounds different to her. She has been taking ibuprofen, which seems to alleviate the headache and body aches but has been ineffective at eliminating the throat pain. Both deny exposure to anyone with similar symptoms. On examination, the patient appears interactive, with a fever recorded at 101.8°F. Her examination is remarkable for tender anterior cervical lymph nodes and erythematous posterior pharynx with a moderate amount of exudate.

APPROACH TO THE PATIENT WITH PHARYNGITIS

When managing pharyngitis in the convenient care setting, there are three primary objectives:

1. Determine the severity of symptoms and rule out clinical emergencies; specifically, assess whether symptoms can be treated in the convenient care setting
2. Determine whether the infection is bacterial or viral in nature and make a diagnosis
3. Define treatment

Determine the Severity of Symptoms and Rule Out Clinical Emergencies

When evaluating a patient with a sore throat, it is important to evaluate the patient's vital signs and clinical picture. Symptoms to watch for include labored breathing, inability to swallow or obvious drooling, swelling of the face or neck, inability to open the mouth, severe pain, asymmetrical swelling of the soft palate, unilateral swelling of the pharynx or tonsils, and deviation of the uvula (Gosselin, 2012). The following are possible diagnoses that require immediate attention and thus cannot be missed.

Epiglottitis

Epiglottitis presents as a toxic-appearing patient with a high fever, stridor, and drooling. The classic description is of a patient leaning forward in a tripod position.

Peritonsillar Abscess

Peritonsillar abscess (PTA) is a potential emergency, because it represents an abscess that forms around the tonsils, potentially leading to an airway obstruction. Patients will usually present with severe sore throat, unilateral throat fullness, and pharyngeal discomfort along with malaise, headaches, and fatigue; some will present with referred ear pain with swallowing, inability to open the mouth, and neck pain (see Figure 4.1). Examination of the oral cavity will show erythema, asymmetry of the soft palate, tonsillar exudate, and displacement of the uvula. In most cases of PTA, treatment is needle aspiration with incision and drainage (I&D), cultures taken, and antibiotic therapy. PTA is a medical emergency that needs to be referred immediately (Gosselin, 2012).

Retropharyngeal Abscess

Patients present with painful swallowing and often have a fever. They may be toxic appearing, and the pharynx may appear full. Retropharyngeal abscess is a

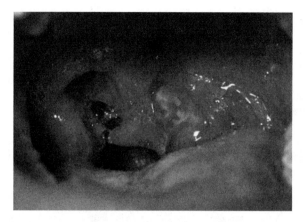

Figure 4.1 ■ Peritonsillar abscess: A bulging tonsil is seen with deviation of the uvula to the opposite side. Note that this will typically require incision and drainage.
(© SPL/Custom Medical Stock Photo)

deep space infection that requires heightened awareness and imaging for detection (Fleisher, 2012, May 9), and usually requires x-ray or CT scan for diagnosis.

It is imperative to recognize these symptoms as medical emergencies and refer these patients immediately to the nearest emergency room for further evaluation and treatment. In addition, dehydrated or septic patients must be referred to a higher level of care. Patients who present with a sore throat at a convenient care clinic (CCC) tend to believe that they have strep throat, but it is the responsibility of the clinician to evaluate and refer as appropriate in case of these rare diagnoses.

Make a Diagnosis

Once you have determined that the patient is appropriate for the convenient care setting, the next step is to determine whether the infection is viral or bacterial in nature. This strategy cannot be underemphasized in the convenient care setting—up to 70% of cases of pharyngitis are viral infections rather than GABHS, which is important in order to limit antibiotic use to appropriate cases. The most common viral causes are rhinovirus and adenovirus. Rare forms of viral pharyngitis include Epstein–Barr virus, cytomegalovirus, herpes simplex virus, respiratory syncytial virus, HIV, parainfluenza, influenza, enterovirus, and coronavirus (Aung, 2011).

There are several approaches to differentiating viral from bacterial pharyngitis in the convenient care setting. Most of these strategies are based on clinical safety and efficacy studies as well as on weighing the cost and side effects of antibiotic treatment. In general, the first test to be used in evaluating a sore throat is the rapid strep test (RST); it should be used as a first-line diagnostic test in all pediatric patients. RST should not be performed on patients who are taking antibiotics, because this may result in a false negative. Despite popular opinion, there are no clinical trials that suggest that RST results can be affected by a patient's eating or drinking beforehand. When taking a swab, it is important not to touch the buccal mucosa or tongue with the swab and to vigorously swab the tonsillar pillars.

In general, an RST can be performed on most patients presenting to a CCC with a chief complaint of sore throat. In some cases, it is appropriate to screen with the Centor score to determine which patients are most appropriate for an RST. All pediatric patients with a chief complaint of a sore throat should undergo an RST.

Centor score: 1 point for each of the following in adult patients. A score of 2 or more is suggestive of a GABHS infection and should have an RST performed.

- Tonsillar exudates
- Cervical adenopathy
- Presence of a fever
- Absence of a cough

When performing an RST, it is important not to touch the tongue, the palate, or the buccal mucosa. Ideal specimens are achieved with vigorous swabbing of both tonsils and the posterior pharynx (Figure 4.2). Two separate swabs should be used if RST and throat cultures are to be performed. The RST swab should not be used for cultures.

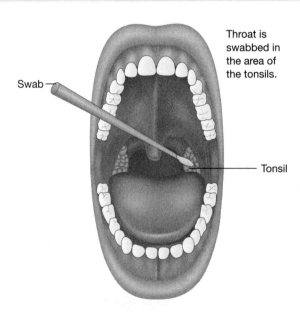

Throat is swabbed in the area of the tonsils.

Swab

Tonsil

Figure 4.2 ■ Proper throat swab technique.

(http://hawaii.gov/health/family-child-health/contagious-disease/influenza/institution_ili/ili_activity_info.htm)

A note on testing: Many national and regional quality reporting organizations measure and report on how many patients are treated without a screening or confirmatory test for GABHS. In the CCC setting, this measures whether providers are empirically treating patients or using evidence-based guidelines. To ensure high quality of care, it is a best practice to test all patients with an RST if antibiotics are to be started. An exception to this rule can be to empirically treat symptomatic family members of a documented GABHS patient.

Although there are many predictive scoring models for pediatrics, there is no scoring methodology that has proven reliable. As such, a good convenient care best practice is to test all pediatrics patients who present with a chief complaint of pharyngitis or in whom there is a clinical suspicion of GABHS. In children, an RST can potentially be avoided when there is a clear viral syndrome (cough, diarrhea, and conjunctivitis). The RST has a specificity of less than 95% and a sensitivity that varies from 65% to 90% (Wald, 2012, September 19). Thus, with a positive RST result, you can confidently treat the patient for GABHS. A negative RST result, however, does not rule out strep throat; in these cases, a throat culture should be considered. Based on well-accepted guidelines, you should send out a throat culture on all pediatric patients with a negative RST.

With adults, because there is a lower probability of complications, cultures need to be ordered only for patients with a higher clinical suspicion of GABHS based on Centor criteria or those who have a personal history of rheumatic heart disease. In the convenient care setting, it is reasonable to send cultures on all patients presenting with sore throats who have a negative RST with a Centor score of +2 and on adults who live with children. This is likely the best strategy to avoid prescribing unnecessary antibiotics and provide a cost-effective and clinically efficient program. Throat cultures are 95% sensitive (Gerber, 1989).

Other bacterial causes of pharyngitis include *Mycoplasma pneumonia*, which accounts for 5% to 16% of cases of pharyngitis in children older than age 6. Rare etiologies include *Neisseria gonorrhoeae* (ask about sexual history), non-Group A streptococci (Group C and G), and *Corynebacterium diphtheria* (hallmarked by the formation of a tightly adhering gray membrane that bleeds when dislodged) (Wald, 2012). Other bacterial pathogens include *Staphylococcus aureus, Haemophilus influenzae, Moraxella catarrhalis, Bacteroides fragilis, Bacteroides oralis, Bacteroides melaninogenicus, Fusobacterium* species, *Peptostreptococcus* species, and, less commonly, *Chlamydia trachomatis* (Simon, 2012).

Differential Diagnosis

Bacterial Pharyngitis

GABHS accounts for 15% to 30% of all cases of pharyngitis in children between the ages of 5 and 15 and up to 30% in adults. The incidence peaks in the winter and early spring because of favorable transmission conditions. Hallmark features of GABHS pharyngitis in addition to a sore throat include abrupt onset of fever, headache, abdominal pain, and nausea or even vomiting; however, neither cough nor significant rhinorrhea is typical for GABHS. It is common to have enlarged tender anterior cervical lymph nodes and an erythematous uvula with tonsillar exudate (Figure 4.3), and, occasionally, a skin rash develops that is known as a scarlatiniform rash (Figure 4.4).

Left untreated, a GABHS infection can lead to suppurative complications such as retropharyngeal abscesses or sinusitis. It can also lead to nonsuppurative or immune-mediated complications such as acute rheumatic fever or acute glomerulonephritis. Most of these complications can be prevented when the infection is

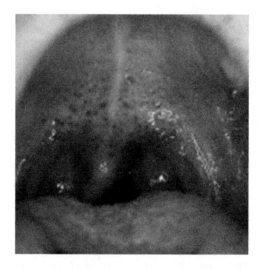

Figure 4.3 ■ Strep pharyngitis: Notice the petechiae and erythema of the posterior pharynx.
(http://hardinmd.lib.uiowa.edu/cdc/3185.html)

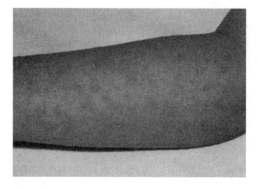

Figure 4.4 ■ Scarlatiniform rash of scarlet fever: A rash of sandpaper-like consistency found occasionally in cases of strep pharyngitis.
(© Science Photo Library/Custom Medical Stock Photo)

treated with antibiotics no later than 9 days after the onset of symptoms. However, to avoid such complications, the accurate diagnosis of GABHS is important.

Viral Pharyngitis

Rhinovirus is responsible for nearly 20% of pharyngitis cases. It does not require antibiotic therapies, although supportive therapies will often help the patient feel better until the virus has run its course. Viral pharyngitis will be the default diagnosis in most cases when bacterial pharyngitis is ruled out.

Laryngitis

Laryngitis is caused by swelling and inflammation of the larynx (voice box) and is usually associated with hoarseness ("Laryngitis," 2010). It is most common in individuals aged 18 to 40 years, affects the membranes that cover the vocal folds, and is typically viral (Shah, 2011). It causes swelling and erythema of the vocal folds; the voice change is a result of the thickening of the entire fold (Shah & Meyers, 2011). Because laryngitis is usually viral in nature, conservative treatment, such as voice rest, decongestants, anti-inflammatories, and humidified air, is enough to improve symptoms until the voice returns to normal ("Laryngitis," 2010).

Mononucleosis

Mononucleosis ("mono") is a viral infection usually accompanied by a sore throat, fever, and swollen lymph nodes, especially in the neck. It is most commonly caused by the Epstein–Barr virus and affects all age groups, although it is more prevalent in those aged 15 to 17 years. It is spread by saliva and is also known as "the kissing disease." Patients may present with sore throat, fever, and swollen nodes but may also complain of fatigue and general malaise. It is also common for patients to present with a prolonged rash or a rash that developed after treatment with amoxicillin. A monospot test should be considered in a patient with these complaints. It is important to remember that it takes 2 weeks of illness to have a positive result; hence, false negatives are common early in the course of the sore throat. Patients can be contagious for up to 4 weeks after symptoms have improved and should also be advised to avoid any type of contact sport due to possible enlargement of the spleen. Treatment goals are primarily related to relief of symptoms ("Mononucleosis," 2012).

Upper Respiratory Infections

Unspecified upper respiratory infections (URIs; the common cold) can be viral or bacterial and the patient can present to the clinic with many different symptoms, including fever, increased nasal drainage, cough, sore throat, and swelling. Treatment for URIs is typically focused on alleviation of symptoms; antibiotics are only clinically indicated for secondary types of infections such as otitis media and sinusitis. Pharyngitis can be caused by influenza, which is characterized by cough, high fever, headache, and body aches; symptoms are typically of sudden onset, and patients may describe feeling "like I was hit by a truck."

TREATMENT

All forms of pharyngitis require symptomatic treatment. Only bacterial pharyngitis requires treatment with antibiotics to prevent complications, reduce transmission and duration, and alleviate symptoms.

Preventing Complications

Possible complications of pharyngitis include nonsuppurative complication such as acute rheumatic fever and suppurative complications such as abscesses. The suppurative complications (sinusitis, abscess, and mastoiditis) can be prevented with antibiotics when the offending pathogen is GABHS. Antibiotics should not be used prophylactically in non-GABHS cases. Nonsuppurative complications include rheumatic fever and glomerulonephritis. Rheumatic fever is an immune-mediated disorder that follows GABHS infections of the throat. It can be significantly reduced when antibiotics are started within 9 days following the onset of symptoms; hence, treatment delay while awaiting culture results is a reasonable strategy. Poststreptococcal glomerulonephritis can follow skin or throat infections but is very rare. There is no evidence that antibiotics can prevent glomerulonephritis (Bisno et al., 2002; Spinks et al., 2006).

Reducing Transmission and Duration

Initiating antibiotics in GABHS cases reduces the rate of transmission by effectively eliminating pharyngeal GABHS within 24 hours.

Decreasing Symptom Severity

Where there are no complications, treatment of pharyngitis is focused on alleviating the severity and duration of the patient's symptoms. When provided in the first 1 to 2 days, antibiotics can decrease the duration of the infection by 1 to 2 days. This highlights the need to also provide symptomatic care.

In general, treatment should be reserved for symptomatic patients with clinical evidence of confirmed GABHS (RST or culture); however, empiric treatment is occasionally required. Empirical treatment can be used for patients with high clinical probability (all four Centor criteria), patients with a personal history of rheumatic heart disease, or patients who have family members or close contacts who were recently diagnosed with GABHS. The rate of transmission among household members can be up to 35%; thus, a reasonable strategy is to treat asymptomatic household contacts in cases where multiple family members are already ill.

First-Line Treatment

Oral penicillin V is the treatment of choice, owing to its proven efficacy, safety, narrow spectrum, and low cost (Pichichero, 2012). Recommended dosing for children is 2 to 50 mg/kg/d four times a day for 10 days and 500 mg two to three times daily for 10 days for adults ("Antibiotics for Strep Throat [Streptococcal Pharyngitis]," 2011). Amoxicillin is often used in place of penicillin V, especially in children, because it is more palatable (Pichichero, 2012). Amoxicillin dosing is 40 mg/kg/d three times a day for 10 days for children and 500 mg three times a day for 10 days for adults ("Antibiotics for Strep Throat," 2011). Intramuscular penicillin G and bicillin are also appropriate for those patients who cannot complete a 10-day course of oral antibiotics or who have a personal history of rheumatic heart disease (Pichichero, 2012).

Second-Line and Recurrent Treatment

Azithromycin and first-generation cephalosporins are also acceptable as therapy in treatment failure with penicillin or amoxicillin or with β-lactam sensitivity (Pichichero, 2012). Common dosing for second-line therapies is as follows:

Augmentin
    Children—40 mg/kg/d two to three times daily for 10 days
    Adults—500 to 875 mg twice a day for 10 days
Erythromycin
    Children—40 mg/kg/d two to four times daily for 10 days
    Adults—400 mg four times a day for 10 days
Azithromycin
    Children—12 mg/kg every day for 5 days or 20 mg/kg every day for 3 days
    Adults—500 mg on day 1 then 250 mg on days 2 to 5
Cephalexin
    Children—25 to 50 mg/kg/d two to four times daily for 10 days
    Adults—500 mg twice a day for 10 days ("Antibiotics for Strep Throat," 2011)

For patients with recurrent strep, multiple antibiotic allergies or intolerance, or history of PTA, a referral for tonsillectomy may be considered. Criteria for consideration include seven or more episodes in the past year, five or more episodes per year in the past 2 years, or three or more episodes per year in the past 3 years, with at least one of the following with each episode: fever greater than 100.9°F, cervical adenopathy, tonsillar exudate, or positive strep test ("Streptococcal Pharyngitis," 2012).

Supportive Therapy

Because over 70% of cases of pharyngitis do not require antibiotics, it is very important that all cases obtain symptomatic support. By taking time to talk to patients about expectations of symptom resolution, and about why antibiotics are not needed, you can avoid antibiotics while ensuring patient satisfaction with care.

The following treatment options can relieve the pain of pharyngitis.

Systemic Therapy

Acetaminophen or nonsteroidal anti-inflammatory drugs (NSAIDs) can be used to help reduce fever, body aches, and headaches and decrease inflammation, which helps to relieve pain. In adults, ibuprofen 400 mg or acetaminophen 1,000 mg can decrease pain perception by at least 50%. Appropriate dosing should be adhered to in pediatrics, and it is helpful to have a guide and instructions to go over with parents. Avoid aspirin and salicylates in pediatrics because of the rare but deadly Reye's syndrome.

Topical Therapy

There are many topical therapies, including lozenges, sprays, and gargles. Despite the presence of many products on the market, there is no one clear superior product. Gargling with salt water can effectively relieve symptoms, although there is no clinical trial to support its efficacy. Lozenges may contain analgesics such as ambroxol, lidocaine, or menthol, and all are effective in reducing pain. Trials have found lozenges with ambroxol, lidocaine, or benzocaine to be more effective than placebo at reducing pain (Stead, 2012). Throat sprays are also thought to be effective and provide better delivery of medication to the posterior pharynx; however, their efficacy has also not been definitely proven in clinical trials.

Corticosteroids

A single dose of dexamethasone at 0.6 mg/kg (max dose 10 mg in children) may hasten improvements in both children and adults, although oral and intramuscular dosing seem to have similar efficacy for relief of symptoms ("Streptococcal Pharyngitis," 2012). Two systematic reviews were done to evaluate dexamethasone 10 mg IM, β-methasone 8 mg IM, and prednisone 60 mg oral. Although all the studies found a decrease in reported pain, these results are somewhat controversial in design. Because of their side-effect profile, it is not recommended that steroids be used routinely in a convenient care setting except in the most severe cases of pain or difficulty swallowing, cases that are also likely better treated in an alternate setting.

Alternative Products

There are no definitive studies that indicate that therapies such as papain, slippery elm, or honey-anise products alleviate pain in pharyngitis. These are best avoided in favor of effective methods.

PATIENT EDUCATION

There are several strategies patients should be encouraged to utilize in order to prevent the further spread of infections, including using tissues to sneeze or cough, washing hands frequently while the infection is active, and not sharing glasses, utensils, or toothbrushes ("Strep Throat," 2011). Encourage patients to increase fluids and rest while they are feeling badly. Advise them that they are considered contagious until they have been on antibiotics for 24 hours and that toothbrushes should either be sterilized or replaced after they are no longer contagious to decrease risk of reinfection ("Streptococcal Pharyngitis," 2012). Patients should see clinical improvement within 3 to 5 days after starting antibiotics or spontaneous resolution by day 5. If a patient fails to improve despite antibiotic use, strongly consider a suppurative complication or a misdiagnosis.

Note: Non–Group A streptococcus (Group C or Group G) can cause a sore throat. These bacteria will not result in a positive RST but may be picked up by throat culture. Because these bacteria do not cause rheumatic fever, their treatment should be focused on alleviating symptoms. When cultures are positive and patients still have symptoms, they can be treated with 5-day courses of antibiotics as they do not cause complications such as rheumatic fever.

Case Resolution: Following evidence-based practice and based on an assessment of the symptoms, the likely diagnosis for the patient is strep throat. An RST confirms with a positive result. As the patient did not appear toxic or dehydrated, it was decided to treat her that day with liquid penicillin and acetaminophen. Her mother was instructed not to use aspirin and to use lozenges for comfort and told how to prevent other family members from getting ill. A note was sent to the patient's pediatrician, and the patient was advised to stay well hydrated.

5

Sinusitis

NIA VALENTINE AND SAMUEL N. GRIEF

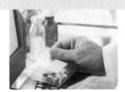

Sinusitis is the symptomatic inflammation of the nasal and paranasal sinuses; the term is used interchangeably with the term rhinosinusitis, because nasal mucosa inflammation usually precedes inflammation of the paranasal sinuses. Annually, approximately one in seven adults develops sinusitis; it is one of the most frequently presenting complaints in the convenient care setting (Pleis, Lucas, & Ward, 2009). The vast majority of cases of sinusitis are viral in nature and represent a component of an upper respiratory tract infection; in only 2% to 5% of cases, the source of the infection is bacterial. One of the primary challenges with treating sinusitis is accurately distinguishing a bacterial infection from a viral one, so that antibiotics are not prescribed needlessly (Fokkens, Lund, & Mullol, 2007).

Case Study: A 26-year-old female patient visits a convenient care clinic (CCC). Her initial complaints include a mild sore throat, postnasal drainage, low-grade fever with maximum temperature of 100.4°F (38.0°C), and a cough starting 10 days ago. Over-the-counter (OTC) multi-symptom medication appeared to have helped—her symptoms only persisted for 5 days and then began to taper off over the next 2 days. Within the past 3 days, however, her symptoms have changed and now she has a headache, nasal congestion, purulent nasal discharge, and facial pain, with no relief from her OTC medication.

DEFINITIONS AND PATHOPHYSIOLOGY

Sinusitis is defined as acute (AS) when symptoms last less than 4 weeks, subacute when symptoms last for 4 to 12 weeks, and chronic when symptoms persist for more than 12 weeks. In general, treatment in the convenient care setting should be limited to acute sinusitis; chronic and subacute cases require imaging and often sinus culturing as well. In addition to determining whether a case is acute, it is also important to try to make a distinction between viral and bacterial sinusitis. Both are caused by inflammation of the nasal and paranasal sinuses by microorganisms, leading to hypersecretion and fluid buildup in the sinus cavities, which then leads to congestion and a sensation of pressure. Almost all cases of sinusitis begin as viral infections, with the primary organisms being rhinovirus, influenza A and B, parainfluenza, respiratory syncytial virus, and enterovirus. Most viral cases of AS will spontaneously improve in 7 to 10 days (Eloy et al., 2011). Occasionally, viral sinusitis can lead to a bacterial superinfection—the sinuses fill with fluid and cannot drain, creating a perfect medium for bacterial growth. These viral infections also impair normal immunity mechanisms, which creates an environment that will lead to bacterial super-infection in 2% to 5% of cases. Where AS has a bacterial cause, common bacteria are *Haemophilus influenzae*, *Moraxella catarrhalis*, *Streptococcus pneumonia*, other *Streptococcus* species, and *Staphylococcus aureus* (Shoup, 2011, 23). Up to one-third of bacterial cases of AS are polymicrobial in nature. Although it is not impossible, it is considered rare to have a bacterial infection within 7 days of onset of symptoms. Thus, if symptom duration is less than 7 days, treatment with antibiotics is rarely indicated (*Health Care Guideline: Diagnosis and Treatment of Respiratory Illness in Children and Adults*, 2011).

APPROACH TO THE PATIENT

Chief Complaint

Many patients presenting to a CCC will present with a chief complaint of "I have a sinus infection" because of their familiarity with the condition. Others will complain of facial pressure, congestion, cough, or runny nose.

History

Critical questions to consider asking the patient to help determine a diagnosis include presentation of symptoms, duration of illness (most vital question), symptom progression, medical history (i.e., allergies, asthma, previous history of AS, smoking habit, compromised immune system, antibiotic use within the past 30 days, olfactory disturbances, and known anatomical blockages).

Review of Symptoms

Common symptoms include facial pressure, nasal drainage, dental pain, halitosis, nasal congestion and rhinorrhea, headache, and cough that worsens at night. A classic description is facial pressure that worsens when the patient bends over. Fever is also a common complaint, although it is usually mild.

Physical Examination

Key components to focus on during the physical examination of a patient with suspected AS are as follows:

- Pay particular attention for the presence of nasal mucosa edema, purulent nasal discharge, and signs of increased nasal blood flow.
- Examine the eyes for periorbital edema or allergic shiners (dark circles under the eyes).
- Palpate the frontal, ethmoid, and maxillary sinuses for tenderness.
- Visually inspect the tympanic membranes for the presence of serous effusions and/or middle-ear infection.
- Examine the pharynx for erythema, postnasal drainage, and lymphoid hypertrophy. Transillumination was once recommended as part of the initial evaluation in cases of suspected AS. Currently, its usefulness is limited and dependent on the provider's skill level, because improper technique can lead to false results (ICSI, 2011). The rest of the physical examination should otherwise be completed normally.
- Sinus pain can also be tested by having the patient bend forward; reproduced or worsening pain is symptomatic of sinusitis. Pain can also be elicited by percussing the upper molars or applying pressure over the frontal or maxillary sinuses (Kogutt & Swischuk, 1973).
- Test all cranial nerves including extraocular motion.

RED FLAGS IN HISTORY OR EXAMINATION

When treating patients in the convenient care setting, it is important to recognize warning signs of conditions requiring immediate referral to another medical facility for urgent or emergent care. These red flags may include any of the following:

- Swelling or redness of the eyelid and periorbital area (preseptal cellulitis)
- Pain with eye movement, inability to move the eye, proptosis, double vision, or loss of vision (orbital cellulitis)
- Fever, headache, nuchal rigidity, altered mental status (meningitis)
- Ptosis, proptosis, limited eye movement, headache, altered mental status, periorbital edema (septic cavernous sinus thrombosis)
- Headache, altered mental status, focal neurological deficit (epidural abscess)
- Urgent referrals should be made for loss of or changes in vision, neurologic symptoms, or altered mental status (Goodhue & Brady, 2004; Eloy et al., 2011; Shoup, 2011). In addition, septic or dehydrated patients will require emergent referral.

DIFFERENTIAL DIAGNOSIS

The symptom of facial pain that may accompany AS is often confused with other possible diagnoses such as viral upper respiratory illness (common cold), allergic rhinitis, tension/stress or migraine headache, dental abscess, foreign body obstruction (nasal polyp or tumor), trigeminal neuralgia, and optic neuritis.

Upper Respiratory Tract Infections

Upper respiratory infections (URIs) often manifest as nasal discharge, nasal congestion, sore throat, and/or cough. Fever may be present in the first few days, usually plateaus at less than 102°F (<39°C), and typically lasts only 24 to 48 hours. It is important to remember that, with the presence of nasal discharge, the clarity, color, or texture of the discharge does not make a bacterial condition more likely. These symptoms are self-limiting within 7 to 10 days and generally follow a similar course of progression and resolution. When symptoms persist more than 10 days or worsen after 5 to 7 days, there is a greater probability of bacterial sinusitis.

Allergic Rhinitis

Allergic rhinitis is an inflammation of the nasal membranes in response to environmental allergens. It is hallmarked by sneezing, congestion, runny nose, and nasal itching that follow a seasonal pattern. The nasal secretions are usually thin and watery. Patients often have a nasal crease from repeated rubbing of the tip of their nose with the palm of their hand. They may also have dark circles around their eyes, also known as "allergic shiners." Treatment involves environmental avoidance and the use of antihistamines and decongestants. An inhaled nasal steroid is often required.

Nasal Foreign Body

Be suspicious when there is unilateral nasal discharge with foul odors.

Dental Abscess

Dental abscesses can usually be determined with a careful oral examination.

Continuation of Case Study: Based on the presenting complaints and the duration, a clinician can confidently state that this is a case of sinusitis. The clinician lets the patient know of the suspected diagnosis and the patient replies, "Just like last year. I knew I needed a Z-pack."

MAKING THE DIAGNOSIS

Acute sinusitis is a clinical diagnosis, and imaging and laboratory evaluation are not required. The primary symptoms that define sinusitis are purulent nasal discharge and nasal congestion or facial pressure. AS presents similarly among pediatric patients, with persistent URI symptoms, daytime cough that is often worse at night, and increasing severity of symptoms over time (Wald, 2012).

One scoring method that has a high predictive value for sinusitis is defined by the Infectious Disease Society of America, which categorizes sinusitis as having two major markers or one major marker and at least two minor markers (Chow et al., 2012) (see Table 5.1). Convenient care clinicians who follow these guidelines will increase the probability of making an accurate diagnosis.

Once diagnosis of sinusitis is made, the next step is to determine whether it is bacterial or viral.

DETERMINING WHETHER SINUSITIS IS BACTERIAL OR VIRAL IN NATURE

Sinusitis can be caused by viruses or bacteria, and in most cases, symptoms for each are similar during the first 7 days, making a clinical diagnosis very difficult. Because the symptoms of viral and bacterial sinusitis are often very similar, the decision to treat with antibiotics is determined by the clinical course (duration and pattern of symptoms) and the severity of the illness.

Table 5.1 ■ Markers for Sinusitis

MAJOR MARKERS	MINOR MARKERS
Purulent nasal discharge	Headache
Purulent postnasal discharge	Ear pain, pressure, and/or fullness
Nasal obstruction or congestion	Sore throat
Facial congestion or fullness	Halitosis
Focal facial pain and/or pressure	Dental pain
Hyposmia or anosmia	Cough
Fever >102°F (39.0°C)	Fever <102°F (39.0°C)
	Fatigue

Source: Modified from Chow et al. (2012).

Viral Sinusitis

Upper respiratory tract infections will usually last 7 to 10 days with gradual improvement throughout the course and with complete resolution by 2 weeks; symptoms usually peak in the first week. Fever is rare, but when it does occur, it is predominantly in the first 1 to 2 days. Symptoms are usually mild to moderate with varying levels of clear or mucopurulent nasal discharge (Wald, 2012).

Bacterial Sinusitis

In general, a diagnosis of bacterial sinusitis is favored by any one of the following (2012 Infectious Disease Society of America Guidelines; Meltzer et al., 2006):

- *Duration of Unremitting Symptoms*: Most viral cases will resolve in 7 to 10 days; thus, cases that last longer than 10 days with persistent, nonimproving symptoms are favored to be bacterial in nature. The most common symptoms to persist will be nasal congestion, presence of a cough that does not improve, and nasal discharge.
- *Pattern*: Symptoms that worsen (new fever, worsening of congestion, or increased amount of nasal discharge) following a period of mild to moderate URI that had been improving—that is, a double sickening—likely indicate a secondary bacterial infection of an original viral sinusitis.
- *Severity*: Severe facial pain, purulent nasal discharge, or fever greater than 39°C or 102°F that has persisted for at least 3 to 4 days at the onset of an illness are predictive of a bacterial infection. Most viral illnesses do not have a high fever, but when they do, the fever lasts just 1 to 2 days.

TREATMENT

Sinusitis treatment has two components: alleviating symptoms and, where applicable, resolving the bacterial infection. All patients presenting with AS should be treated for symptom alleviation.

Symptomatic Treatment

All patients who present with symptoms of sinusitis should be treated with analgesia. Many will benefit from inhaled glucocorticoids.

- *Fever and Pain Control*: All patients presenting with acute sinusitis should receive analgesia nonsteroidal anti-inflammatory drugs and acetaminophen, although aspirin should be avoided in pediatric patients because of the potential risk for developing Reye's syndrome.

- *Saline Irrigation*: Clinical evidence supports the use of saline irrigation with hypertonic saline to reduce symptoms associated with sinusitis (Kassel, King, & Spurling, 2010).
- *Intranasal Steroids*: Topical steroids work to decrease inflammation in the nasal and paranasal sinuses. Many studies have found differing levels of efficacy, but steroids are suggested by many authorities and may be useful in treating associated nasal congestion and sinus pressure, particularly in patients with allergic rhinitis as a complicating factor (Meltzer, Teper, & Danzig, 2008; Small et al., 2007).
- *Topical/Oral Decongestants*: The theoretical use of decongestants is to reduce edema and increase drainage of the sinuses. There are no studies that demonstrate a clear benefit and their use should be limited. Avoid decongestants in patients with uncontrolled hypertension, hyperthyroidism, coronary artery disease, diabetes, glaucoma, and benign prostatic hypertrophy. Use of topical decongestants should be limited to no more than 3 days to lessen the risk of rebound nasal congestion.
- *Antihistamines*: Similar to decongestants, antihistamines have a theoretical role in reducing tissue edema. However, they also increase the viscosity of secretions, decrease blood flow to the nasal mucosa, and can impair sinus drainage (Wald, 2012).

Antimicrobial Treatment

When bacterial sinusitis is suspected, antibiotics are warranted. Antibiotics are used to shorten the duration of acute bacterial rhinosinusitis (ABRS), decrease transmission, reduce the probability of complications, and relieve symptoms. Antibiotic choice should be oriented toward eradicating the most commonly cultured bacteria and recognizing the increase in antimicrobial resistance to amoxicillin in pneumococci and *H. influenzae* (resistance rates vary by region but are as high as 60% in some areas). Updated treatment guidelines recommend amoxicillin-clavulanate (Augmentin) rather than amoxicillin alone as the empiric first-line choice for acute sinusitis in both adults and children (Chow et al., 2012). Macrolides (clarithromycin and azithromycin) are not recommended for empiric therapy because of high rates of resistance among *S. pneumoniae* (~30%). March 12, 2013, the Food and Drug Administration issued new warnings regarding azithromycin use, which could lead to potentially fatal irregular heart rhythm, and should be heeded as necessary. Trimethoprim-sulfamethoxazole is not recommended for empiric therapy because of high rates of resistance among both *S. pneumoniae* and *H. influenzae* (~30%–40%). Doxycycline may be used as an alternative regimen to amoxicillin-clavulanate for initial empiric antimicrobial therapy of ABRS in adults, because it remains highly active against respiratory pathogens and has excellent pharmacokinetic/pharmacodynamic properties.

Second- and third-generation oral cephalosporins are no longer recommended for empiric monotherapy of ABRS because of variable rates of resistance among *S. pneumoniae*. Combination therapy with a third-generation oral cephalosporin (cefixime or cefpodoxime) plus clindamycin may be used as second-line therapy for children with non–type I penicillin allergy or from geographic regions with high endemic rates of penicillin-nonsusceptible *S. pneumonia* (PNS).

Either doxycycline (not suitable for children) or a respiratory fluoroquinolone (levofloxacin or moxifloxacin) is recommended as an alternative agent for empiric antimicrobial therapy in adults who have moderate or strong allergic reactions to penicillin.

Levofloxacin is recommended for children older than age 8 with a history of type I hypersensitivity to penicillin; combination therapy with clindamycin plus a third-generation oral cephalosporin (cefixime or cefpodoxime) is recommended in children with a history of non–type I hypersensitivity to penicillin (see Table 5.2).

The recommended duration of therapy for uncomplicated ABRS in adults is 5 to 7 days. In children with acute bacterial sinusitis, the longer treatment duration of 10 to 14 days is still recommended (Wald, 2012).

If symptoms have not improved by the completion of the first-line antibiotic, a second-line antibiotic should be used. Empiric second-line antibiotics

Table 5.2 ■ Recommended Antibiotics

	ADULTS	PEDIATRICS
First line	Amoxicillin-clavulanate 500 mg/125 mg po tid or 875 mg/125 mg po bid	Amoxicillin-clavulanate 45 mg/kg bid of the amoxicillin or 90 mg/kg bid if the child has had antibiotics in the last 30 days, attends day care, or is <2 years of age
First line	Augmentin 2 g po bid In immunocompromised adults or those over age 65, on antibiotics within the last 30 d, with severe disease (fever >39°C or 102°F), or in areas with high PCN resistance	Use high dose with patients from a geographic region with high endemic rates (≥10%) of invasive PNS, severe infection (e.g., evidence of systemic toxicity with fever of 39°C [102°F] or higher, threat of suppurative complications), attendance at daycare, age <2, recent hospitalization, antibiotic use within the past month, or with immunocompromised (weak, moderate) status
PCN allergy type I	Avelox 400 mg po qd Doxycycline 100 mg po bid Levofloxacin 500 mg po qd	Levofloxacin 10 to 20 mg/kg/d divided every 12 or 24 hours
PCN allergy non-type I		Cefpodoxime 10 mg/kg/d orally divided every 12 hours or cefdinir 14 mg/kg per day orally divided every 12 or 24 hours

PNS, penicillin-nonsusceptible *S. pneumonia*; PCN, penicillin.
Source: Hwang and Getz (2012).

include amoxicillin-clavulanate 2,000 mg/125 mg orally twice daily (90 mg/kg in pediatrics orally twice daily), levofloxacin 500 mg orally every day, or moxifloxacin 400 mg orally every day. Patients who do not respond to the second-line antibiotics should be referred to an otolaryngologist to further investigate the refractory symptoms.

RECOMMENDED DISPOSITION AND PATIENT EDUCATION

Patient education is the key to successfully treat AS. Patients should be aware that URI and acute viral sinusitis mimic each other initially and that antibiotic use is neither warranted nor beneficial with those diagnoses.

Reinforce to patients the differences between acute viral sinusitis and acute bacterial sinusitis in order to reassure and lessen unrealistic expectations vis-à-vis antibiotic use. It is important to discuss when to use comfort measures and when to seek medical treatment. A number of sources for patients discuss comfort measures; however, providers should supply a list of adequate home self-care measures, which may include (1) maintain adequate hydration (6 to 10 glasses of liquids per day to thin mucus); (2) humidify the home environment; (3) apply warm facial packs (warm washcloth, hot water bottle, or gel pack for 5 to 10 minutes three or more times a day to help with pain relief); (4) eliminate environmental factors that could trigger allergic reactions (cigarette smoke, pollution or fumes, swimming in contaminated water, barotraumas); (5) obtain adequate rest and sleep with head of bed elevated; (6) avoid extremely cold or dry air; and (7) engage in fastidious and frequent hand washing (ICSI, 2011). These measures will likely decrease the number of patients that need to be treated with antibiotics for acute bacterial sinusitis.

Any patient with a red flag should be emergently referred to an ER for imaging. Patients with more than three or four episodes a year should be referred nonemergently to an ENT physician.

Case Resolution: The 26-year-old female's case presentation meets the diagnostic criteria for ABS based on her biphasic symptoms of headache, nasal congestion, purulent nasal discharge, and facial pain that followed after a typical viral infection of 5 days with 2 days of improving symptoms. She was given the first-line antibiotic of amoxicillin 500 mg two tablets every 8 hours for 7 days.

6

Cough and Upper Respiratory Tract Infections

JOSHUA RIFF AND SANDRA F. RYAN

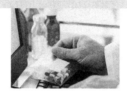

Symptoms of an acute upper respiratory tract infection (URI) and a chief complaint of cough are common presentations at a convenient care clinic (CCC). Twenty percent of convenient care visits come from complaints of cough (Murphy & Williams, 2010), and it is one of the top five conditions seen by CCC providers. Approximately 10 in every 1,000 outpatient visits per year are for complaints of cough, representing close to 30 million visits (Cherry, Burt, & Woodwell, 2011). Although most URIs are benign in origin, the symptoms are deemed quite disruptive and have great impact on productivity and quality of life.

Case Study: A 39-year-old female complains of fatigue and persistent cough for 6 days. The cough has gotten worse over the past 2 days, and she reports that it is most severe at night when she is lying down. The patient experienced sudden onset of fever, chills, profuse runny nose, and myalgia 6 days ago. On the first day of illness, she left work at a local middle school where she is employed as a physical education instructor. Most of her symptoms have resolved, but the cough and fatigue remain. She has been taking over-the-counter (OTC) dextromethorphan and guaifenesin with little to no improvement in her symptoms.

PATHOPHYSIOLOGY AND EPIDEMIOLOGY OF A COUGH

Cough is a reflex that is initiated by bronchial irritation and triggered by the release of inflammatory compounds in lung tissue in response to a foreign body such as viruses or bacteria (Campbell & Super, 2003). Inflammation triggers the cough reflex arc by activating the cough receptors, which ascend through the vagus nerve to the medulla; the efferent signal then travels down the vagus, phrenic, and spinal motor nerves to expiratory musculature to produce the cough as a protective mechanism to forcefully expel foreign material from the lungs.

Inflammation initiated by infectious etiology can overwhelm the natural immune system. In response to infection, the cells releases cytokines, which attract polymorphonuclear cells (PMNs). As the amount of PMNs increase, the thickness of respiratory secretions changes; as the PMNs become more enzymatically active, secretion color changes to green. Hence, the consistency, volume, and color of secretions do not correlate to the etiology being viral or bacterial but instead represent a nonspecific inflammatory response.

APPROACH TO THE PATIENT WITH A COUGH

History

Key components of patient history that help diagnose the etiology of the cough include duration, severity, and associated symptoms. Duration of the cough is key to distinguish acute cough from chronic. In general, coughs lasting less than 3 weeks are considered acute coughs, 3- to 8-week coughs are subacute, and coughs lasting longer than 8 weeks are defined as chronic. Subacute and chronic coughs usually require imaging and, occasionally, specialist referral.

Medical history is also important to review, because some features, such as a history of congestive heart failure or HIV, will complicate the ability to diagnose and treat a cough in a convenient care setting without imaging technology. Medical history that includes chronic lung disease or immunosuppressive states can complicate the care of a patient with a URI. In addition, social history (cigarette use) and medication list (angiotension-converting enzyme [ACE] inhibitors can cause cough) review are important.

Review of Systems

Patients presenting with URIs should be asked about systemic symptoms including fever and myalgias. Also ask about respiratory status and symptoms of wheezing or shortness of breath. Weight loss or night sweats are also pertinent questions to ask.

Physical Examination

The goal of the physical examination is to document a general impression of the patient. Is he or she speaking in full sentences? Is he or she having difficulty breathing? Does the patient appear anxious? One key component with a complaint of cough is auscultation of the lungs—you are listening for rales, crackles (fluid buildup suggestive of congestive heart failure), and wheezing (airway restriction in asthma or chronic obstructive pulmonary disease [COPD]). In addition, it is beneficial to look at the patient's legs for pitting edema, which is suggestive of congestive heart failure (CHF). Respiratory rate and hemoglobin saturation levels should be obtained in all patients, including children. Lastly, document in your note whether cough is present during the examination and, if so, its nature.

RED FLAGS

Emergent referrals are needed when a patient has concerning findings and difficulty breathing or has symptoms suggesting diagnoses beyond the scope of a CCC. In general,

- Patients showing signs of respiratory distress or active asthma will require urgent follow-up.
- Symptoms persisting for more than 3 weeks suggest a chronic cough, which would require further evaluation and treatment. Imaging is often needed when a cough has persisted more than 3 weeks. Each CCC should have established policies on management of these types of patients.
- Harsh, barking, seal-like cough in a child suggests croup, which requires bronchodilators and steroids.
- High fever in a toxic-appearing patient can suggest pneumonia or SARS.
- Night sweats, weight loss, or hemoptysis can be indicators for cancer or TB.
- Recent travel or surgery and/or history of hypercoagulable state put a patient at high risk for pulmonary embolism.
- Whooping-type cough or a high-pitched noise when breathing is suggestive of whooping cough in a young child.
- A patient presenting with signs and symptoms of a URI with a cough who also has a fever, abnormal vital signs, and consolidation on auscultation has a high probability of having pneumonia. It is not generally considered a best practice to make a clinical diagnosis of pneumonia without x-ray confirmation; thus, these patients should have an x-ray ordered or be referred to a higher level of care.

Continuation of Case Study: The physical examination reveals a patient in apparently healthy condition, well nourished, and hydrated, in no acute distress, with normal vital signs. She appears comfortable and is speaking in full sentences. A respiratory examination reveals no wheezing, crackles, rhonchi, or rales. The patient's chest expands symmetrically with normal breath sounds and is clear bilaterally.

The presence of the findings listed below suggests that an x-ray should be obtained.

- Heart rate greater than 100 bpm
- Respiratory rate greater than 24 breaths per minute
- Oral temperature greater than 38°C/100.4°F
- Chest examination suggestive of focal consolidation; egophony or fremitus

They should also be obtained for patients with low pulse oxygen assessment, altered mental status, or toxic-appearing patients. Some clinicians would also recommend a chest x-ray in any elderly patient with a cough.

DIFFERENTIAL DIAGNOSIS

The first step after determining that the patient is stable and appropriate for care in a CCC is to establish the duration of cough. The American College of Chest Physicians (ACCP) defines an acute cough as one lasting less than 3 weeks. The majority of coughs lasting less than 3 weeks will be secondary to an acute or resolving infectious process. Coughs lasting more than 3 weeks may also be related to an infectious process, but in general, unless an obvious cause is evident, these cases should include a chest x-ray as part of the initial workup. Our differential diagnosis will focus on the evaluation and treatment of acute cough.

After defining the cough as acute or chronic, the next step in evaluating the cough is to distinguish between infectious and noninfectious etiologies.

Noninfectious Differential Diagnosis of Cough

Upper Airway Cough Syndrome: Previously known as postnasal drip, upper airway cough syndrome (UACS) can cause subacute or chronic cases of cough. This may be secondary to allergies or a postinfectious cause. The clues to this diagnosis are the sensation of liquid dripping in the back of the throat and a cobblestone appearance of the posterior pharynx. These patients report a constant need to clear their throat. Their cough often increases at night when lying down.

Asthma: Cough may be the sole manifestation of asthma. This is usually diagnosed by a specialist after empiric treatment for cough or UACS has failed.

Gastroesophageal Reflux: Cough can occasionally be the only symptom related to gastroesophageal reflux disease (GERD). Similar to asthma, this diagnosis in absence of classic GERD symptoms is usually made after a failed empiric trial by a specialist.

ACE Inhibitors: A nonproductive cough in a patient on ACE inhibitors (ACE-I) should be considered ACE-I-related until proven otherwise; 15% of patients on ACE-Is will have this side effect (Silvestri & Weinberger, 2011). The cough usually begins a week after starting therapy but can be delayed up to 6 months.

Allergies: Consider seasonal allergies when a seasonal pattern exists. These patients should empirically be started on outpatient allergy medications.

Infectious Differential Diagnosis

The Common Cold

Accounting for 25 million medical visits per year, the common cold is the number-one reason for CCC visits. A cold is a self-limiting viral infection with the primary pathogen being rhinovirus, followed by adenovirus, influenza and parainfluenza virus, and respiratory syncytial virus (RSV); however, over 200 viruses have been implicated. The common cold peaks in the fall and winter months and is transmitted primarily though hand contact—cold-inducing viruses can remain viable on human skin for up to 2 hours (Sexton & McClain, 2011). On average, a child younger than 6 years old will have six to eight colds per year, with each episode lasting 14 days. Older children and adults will have two to four colds per year lasting 5 to 7 days each (Hendley, 1998). Primary symptoms include cough, sneezing, congestion, rhinorrhea, sore throat, headache, and malaise. Fever is common in children but less frequent in adults. A common cold often follows a distinct pattern of symptoms. The first day is usually hallmarked by a sore or scratchy throat (Tyrrell, Cohen, & Schlarb, 1993). The second day is predominated by nasal symptoms including nasal congestion, sneezing, and rhinorrhea. A cough becomes predominant on the fourth or fifth day of the illness, at which time the nasal symptoms begin to diminish (Sexton & McClain, 2011; Tyrrell et al., 1993). The cough is frequently the most bothersome complaint and usually improves after 1 to 2 weeks. When symptoms fail to greatly improve or resolve by 2 weeks, other diagnoses should be considered. Other signs or symptoms that suggest a different etiology include a high persistent fever, focal consolidation on lung examination, or absence of rhinorrhea or nasal congestion. A diagnosis of common cold is usually made clinically when sinusitis and pharyngitis are ruled out clinically or with diagnostic tests.

Bronchitis

Acute bronchitis is inflammation of the upper bronchi; it is most often secondary to a virus and is self-limiting. The majority of patients with bronchitis present with a chief complaint of a cough that lasts for more than 5 days. Left untreated, bronchitis will usually resolve on its own in 1 to 3 weeks. The most important lesson for CCC practitioners is that this illness does not require antibiotics for treatment. Despite this knowledge, 60% to 90% of patients presenting with bronchitis will be prescribed antibiotics (File, 2012). Antibiotics are unnecessary because the most common pathogens—including rhinovirus, influenza, parainfluenza, coronavirus, and RSV—are viral and will not respond to antibacterial treatment. Bacteria can occasionally cause bronchitis—the most common agents are *Mycoplasma pneumoniae*, *Chlamydia pneumoniae*, and pertussis. Of these, only pertussis requires antimicrobial treatment.

Acute bronchitis is indistinguishable from a URI at the onset of illness; however, when cough persists beyond 5 days, acute bronchitis should be considered (Wenzel & Fowler, 2006). Fever is rare in bronchitis (and when present is usually low), and its presence should increase concern for pneumonia or influenza. Patients with bronchitis have few constitutional signs or symptoms beyond the first few days of illness, and the cough will usually last for 10 to 20 days. On physical examination, the patient may have rhonchi but should not have signs of pulmonary consolidation, suggesting pneumonia. The sputum produced during coughing may be purulent, green, and copious, which also does not signal a bacterial infection. Occasionally, bronchitis can cause airway hyperreactivity, which will present as wheezing that sounds like asthma. This wheezing will usually resolve in the course of a month. Although the diagnosis is clinical, influenza testing should be used when clinical suspicion exists.

Pneumonia

When a cough presents with constitutional signs including ill-appearing patients, high fever, or abnormal vital signs (tachypnea or tachycardia), or when the physical examination demonstrates signs of focal pulmonary consolidation, a chest x-ray should be pursued to rule out pneumonia.

Influenza

Influenza is a significant infection caused by the influenza A or B viruses. These infections are hallmarked by upper and lower respiratory symptoms along with systemic illness. Infection usually manifests as a severe illness with an abrupt onset of fever, a cough with significant myalgias, and headache, in addition to rhinitis and a sore throat. It is also usually accompanied by a high fever (>39.0°C or 102.2°F). The physical examination is usually unremarkable, and focal signs of pneumonia should be carefully ruled out. The diagnosis is predominantly made clinically, and testing is not needed when high cases of influenza are being detected in the community. Most CCCs will utilize rapid antigen tests, which have poor sensitivity and high specificity. A good approach for convenient care clinicians is to use clinical criteria alone for diagnosis during times of high community prevalence. In cases where a clinician is uncertain of the diagnosis or when influenza rates are low in the community, influenza rapid antigen testing is a reasonable screening mechanism. The interpretation of the test should be guided by the prevalence of influenza in the community. When prevalence is high, a positive screen is likely a true positive; however, a negative rapid test in a patient with symptoms is likely a false negative. During times of low circulation, a positive test is likely negative and should have a confirmatory test, whereas a negative is likely a true negative. Hence, if you clinically believe a patient has influenza and will require treatment, you should treat regardless of the results of the test. If your pretest probability is low, then it is worthwhile to test and treat only if the rapid test is positive. Prevalence rates should be followed at a clinic level and are available through the Centers for Disease Control and Prevention and the World Health Organization. Patients who are at higher risk of influenza complications (>65, pregnant, chronic lung disease including asthma, heart disease, immunosuppressed, or morbidly obese) should undergo testing if clinical suspicion is low enough not to start empiric therapy but prevalence is high—these patients have the greatest benefit from initiation of antiviral therapy. All patients should be treated with symptomatic care. Patients at high risk of complications may receive antivirals. Each clinic should have a developed policy regarding which patients should be treated with which drugs.

Mycoplasmic Lower Respiratory Tract Infections

These infections present with a slow, smoldering, harsh, dry cough worsening over a period of 3 weeks, predominately in ages 5 to 20 years. This diagnosis is usually made when bronchitis fails to improve or during times of high community infection or known epidemics.

TREATMENT

One of the challenges in treating patients with cough is managing expectations— roughly 90% of cough cases are caused by viruses, yet the majority of Americans today are improperly treated with antibiotics when they are diagnosed with bronchitis. When antibiotics are not required, the greatest tool you have at your disposal is educating patients and managing their symptoms. Hence, when treating patients with signs of URIs including cough, there are three important steps:

Step 1: Manage the patient's expectations and educate the patient
Step 2: Provide symptomatic relief
Step 3: Provide targeted treatment when possible

Managing Expectations and Patient Education

Reassurance and education regarding the natural progression of viral upper and lower airway infection are key starting points. Clearly articulate to patients that they can expect the symptoms of most respiratory illnesses to resolve within a week to 11 days. In addition, some clinicians report that using a term such as "chest cold" provides more reassurance than a term such as bronchitis. It is also important to make sure that parents understand warning signs and when to return to the CCC or to their primary care physician's (PCP's) office.

Symptomatic Care

There are many different drugs and modalities used to manage the symptoms of URI and cough. Choices should be made based on the patient's most bothersome symptoms. A good technique is to ask a patient, "if there is one symptom you would want eliminated, what would it be?" A vital therapeutic modality is hydration. Maintaining adequate hydration allows for the thinning of the mucosa, which allows for better clearance. Ingestion of warm fluids can loosen respiratory secretions. Other treatments to relieve symptoms include those that follow.

Topical Saline

Nasal sprays and bulb suctioning are a valuable method for removing nasal secretions and increase symptomatic relief.

Honey

In children older than 1 year, honey has a beneficial effect in diminishing cough; 1 teaspoon used as needed helps to diminish symptoms associated with URI.

Lozenges

Lozenges seem to work by coating the throat and diminishing cough receptors.

NSAIDs

Many patients with URIs will benefit from a course of nonsteroidal anti-inflammatory drugs (NSAIDs) or acetaminophen. These are proven effective for fever and systemic symptoms.

Cough Suppressants

Decrease the discomfort associated with a frequent cough by suppressing the cough reflex. The ACCP guidelines do not recommend using a cough suppressant for acute cough associated with a URI or acute bronchitis, based on the fact that no study has conclusively found that codeine or dextromethorphan decrease cough symptoms (Bolser 2006).

Decongestants

In theory, decongestants constrict blood flow to the mucosa, leading to less congestion. OTC drugs such as pseudoephedrine and phenylephrine are common active ingredients in oral decongestants, and drugs such as oxymetazoline are used in topical preparations. These drugs may be effective in decreasing symptoms associated with nasal congestion in patients younger than age 12. They should be used sparingly in patients with heart disease, as they frequently cause tachycardia, palpitations, and elevated blood pressure. Topical decongestants should not be used for more than 2 to 3 days due to the risk of rebound rhinitis.

Antihistamines

Diphenhydramine, chlorpeniramine, brompheniramine, doxylamine, and others work through anticholinergic pathways to decrease nasal congestion but have a high side-effect profile (sedation, hallucinations, and respiratory depression). In general, they should be avoided in children younger than age 12 and in older adults.

Ipratropium

0.06% nasal spray tid can be helpful to relieve symptoms associated with excessive and persistent rhinorrhea or sneezing. Side effects include nosebleeds and mouth dryness.

Inhaled (Topical) Nasal Glucocorticoids

Fluticasone or beclomethasone may be helpful in acute rhinosinusitis by decreasing inflammation and subjective symptoms of congestion. They are rarely helpful for rhinorrhea and should be avoided in pediatrics.

Targeted Therapy

M. pneumonia

Nearly 5% of acute coughs are mycoplasmic in nature (Gilbert, Moellering, Eliopoulos, Saag, & Chambers, 2011). In general, this condition is indistinguishable from bronchitis and does not warrant testing or empiric treatment unless a community outbreak exists. *Mycoplasma* and *Chlamydia pneumoniae* are sensitive to tetracycline and fluoroquinolones.

Pertussis

During outbreaks, pertussis can be treated with erythromycin or azithromycin.

Influenza

Antiviral therapy within the first 24 to 48 hours can help shorten the duration of flu symptoms as well as decrease the severity and incidence of complications. Treatment is usually based on the neuraminidase inhibitors—oral oseltamivir and inhaled zanamivir. In general, individuals with severe disease or at high risk of complications should be treated with antivirals. Signs of high risk include (Zachary, 2012):

- Patients older than age 65
- Pregnant women and women up to 2 weeks postpartum
- Patients with chronic pulmonary disease, including asthma
- Chronic cardiovascular disease, excluding hypertension
- Chronic renal or liver disease
- Diabetes mellitus

- Immunosuppression, including cancer
- Any neurological condition that can compromise handling of respiratory secretions (e.g., seizure disorder and spinal cord injuries)
- Morbid obesity

Patients younger than 65 who are not high risk and who present more than 48 hours after onset should not be treated with antivirals, because the side effects outweigh the benefits. If patients present within 48 hours, treatment can be helpful in decreasing the severity and duration of symptoms. As resistance patterns and circulating strains change each year, CCC management should create annual updates, guidelines, and checklists to guide treatment decisions.

Other Treatments

There is a lack of data to support the use of codeine, dextromethorphan, or inhaled β-2-agonists in cases of bronchitis. In general, antibiotics do not have a role in treating acute bronchitis. Consideration for antibiotics can be made for patients older than age 65, with two or more of the following:

- Admission to hospital in the previous year
- Diabetes mellitus
- History of congestive heart failure
- Current use of oral glucocorticoids

In addition, patients at risk of serious complications due to immunosuppression or chronic heart or lung disease may be considered for antimicrobial therapy. Ipratropium can be helpful in treating the cough associated with bronchitis.

The Common Cold

The primary tenets of treating the common cold are to set expectations (in younger children, symptoms can last 14 days; most adults will improve by day 7) and provide supportive care. This includes hydration, humidified air, and ingestion of warm fluids. OTC medications are not recommended for children younger than age 6. Most patients would benefit from relief with acetaminophen or ibuprofen. Ipratropium may have a role in treating excessive rhinorrhea. Cromolyn sodium (intranasal) may help decrease the duration of the common cold when provided as a nasal spray (5.2 mg per spray).

DISPOSITION

Patients who do not improve or worsen, who have subjective shortness of breath and dehydration, should be considered for further workup, including radiographic studies and pertussis screening with a PCP, urgent care center, or emergency department depending on severity of symptoms, location, and availability of higher levels of medical care.

Case Resolution: The patient started with symptoms suggestive of influenza. However, as cough is her predominant symptom and it has persisted for more than 5 days, she most likely has bronchitis. There are no findings suggestive of pneumonia, and she is a good candidate for outpatient therapy. It was recommended that she stop taking the codeine and she was prescribed ipratropium for 5 days with instructions to follow up with her PCP should her symptoms fail to resolve within 10 days.

7

Dysuria and Urinary Complaints

SANGEETHA LARSEN AND AUGUSTINE SOHN

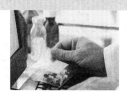

Case Study: A 30-year-old female presents with 3 days of increased urinary frequency and burning sensation with urination. She is sexually active and has been with the same partner for the past 2 years. She denies any history of sexually transmitted diseases (STDs) or any known exposure to them. She denies any fever, chills, nausea, vomiting, flank pain, or abdominal pain. She has not noted any unusual color or odor to her vaginal discharge, and she denies any itching or rashes in the genital region. Of note, she had an episode of pyelonephritis 4 months ago, and she usually gets about one or two urinary tract infections (UTIs) a year. She is not pregnant or breastfeeding. She takes birth control pills but no other medicine, and she has no known drug allergies.

Her vitals are all normal, and a physical examination is unremarkable. A dipstick shows moderate leukocyte estrase, no nitrites, moderate blood, negative protein, pH 6.5, negative ketones, and negative glucose.

EPIDEMIOLOGY AND PATHOPHYSIOLOGY

UTIs are most common in adult females, accounting for approximately 7 million episodes of cystitis (infection ascends to involve the kidneys) and 250,000 episodes of pyelonephritis (infection of the bladder) per year in the United States (Hooton & Stamm, 1997). In pregnancy, UTI incidence is 8% (Delzell & Lefevre, 2000). UTIs affect 2.4% to 2.8% of all children annually (White, 2011). The prevalence of UTIs in young men is equal to or less than 0.1% and 10% in men 65 years old or older (Brusch, 2011).

Most UTIs occur when fecal flora colonize the vaginal introitus, ascend the urethra, and multiply in the bladder. Because of their straighter, shorter urethras, women are more commonly infected than men. Men have both a longer urethra and a drier periurethra, as well as an antibacterial substance in their prostatic fluid; all these combine to make UTIs rarer in men. Infection that ascends the ureter can involve the kidneys, setting the stage for pyelonephritis. *Escherichia coli* is the inciting organism in up to 95% of UTIs; other etiologies include *Proteus mirabilis* and *Klebsiella pneumonia*.

APPROACH TO THE PATIENT WITH URINARY COMPLAINTS

History

There are several important questions to ask when approaching a patient with a urinary complaint (Bremnor & Sadovsky, 2002).

- *Duration*: How long have symptoms been present? Symptoms lasting more than 7 days typically indicate a complicated UTI.
- *Severity*: Is the pain mild, moderate, or severe?
- *Timing*: When does the pain occur? Patients with UTIs usually have a burning sensation during urination and may also generally have pain in the flank or suprapubic areas.
- *Localization*: Is the pain limited to the urethra, or does the patient have pain in the flank areas, abdomen, testes, and so on?
- *Frequency*: How frequently does the patient feel symptoms?
- *Nocturia*: Is the patient wetting the bed at night? This may be a behavioral issue in children or may be a sign of diabetes in either children or adults.
- *Hematuria*: Has the patient noticed any blood in the toilet or when wiping? This may be associated with a UTI, kidney stones, or cancer of the urinary tract, but a female patient could also be having her menses at the same time as the infection.
- *Discharge*: Has the patient experienced any discharge with unusual color or odor? This can indicate a yeast infection in women or an STD in either sex.
- *Last menstrual period*: If a female patient's last menses was over a month before the examination, consider the possibility of pregnancy; pregnancy can predispose women to UTIs.
- *Sexual activity*: In younger men, UTI is often associated with a history of anatomical abnormality. In the absence of evidence of abnormality, collect a detailed sexual history—new or multiple sexual partners and other risk-taking behaviors can be associated with STD-related urethritis, prostatitis, and epididymitis. Patients may be reluctant to reveal a full and accurate history, hence, maintain a high degree of suspicion.

- *Prior related symptoms and infections*: Is there a history of known urinary tract abnormalities, incontinence, or previous UTIs? Ask elderly men about a history of prostatic enlargement, urinary dribbling or hesitancy, or difficulty initiating the urinary stream.
- *New products*: Has the patient introduced any new detergents, personal hygiene products, bubble baths, or spermicides?

Most UTIs in adult women are considered uncomplicated and will respond to basic treatment. However, complications are possible that can prolong the illness or encourage antibiotic resistance because of overuse. Below are factors that can contribute to complicated UTIs. If physical examination or patient history reveals any of these factors, sending out a urine culture for testing may be warranted and a longer treatment period may be called for (ICSI, 2006).

- Symptoms lasting 7 days or more
- Pregnancy
- Diabetes mellitus
- Immunosuppression
- Male patient
- History of renal calculi, renal insufficiency, or renal transplant
- Three or more UTIs in the past year
- Failure of UTI treatment within the past 4 weeks
- Hospital-acquired UTI
- Acute pyelonephritis in the last year
- Indwelling catheter or urinary tract instrumentation within the past 2 weeks
- Functional or anatomic abnormality of the urinary tract
- Antimicrobial use within the past month
- History of recurrent UTIs in childhood
- Younger than 18 or older than 65 (*Note*: It is unclear whether advanced age alone increases the risk of a complicated infection, and few studies have evaluated shorter antibiotic courses in older patients [Mehnert-Kay, 2005]. Providers should use their own judgment to decide if otherwise healthy women older than 65 years with uncomplicated infections can be treated for only 3 days or whether a longer course is indicated.)

It is important to collect and assess all historical features that could indicate a complicated cystitis; without longer treatment and/or stronger antibiotics, complicated infections can lead to sepsis, renal abscesses, and emphysematous pyelonephritis.

Review of Systems

Typical symptoms of a UTI may include any of the following: dysuria, urinary frequency, urgency, hesitancy, incomplete voids, hematuria, and suprapubic or low back pain. Of note, it is important to be particularly suspicious when evaluating children, because fever may be the only presenting complaint (White, 2011). Pyelonephritis should be suspected when symptoms include fever higher than 38°C, chills, flank pain, and systemic symptoms like nausea and vomiting.

Physical Examination

In addition to collecting patient history, the provider should conduct a thorough physical examination, including taking vital signs and checking for abdominal or costovertebral angle (CVA) tenderness. Providers should also look for symptoms outside of the genitourinary tract, such as joint swelling (seen in Behcet's disease), conjunctival erythema (seen with gonococcal conjunctivitis), and oral lesions or rashes (which may be seen with an STD). With complaints that are suggestive of vaginitis, pelvic examinations may also be helpful (Bent, Nallamothu, Simel, Fihn, & Saint, 2002; Bremnor & Sadovsky, 2002).

Red Flags

The following symptoms or signs are suggestive of acute pyelonephritis (Bent et al., 2002; Bremnor & Sadovsky, 2002):

- Fever higher than 100.4°F, chills, nausea, and/or vomiting
- Moderate to severe suprapubic or abdominal tenderness
- Moderate to severe unilateral or bilateral CVA tenderness

Different clinics may allow for outpatient treatment of acute *uncomplicated* pyelonephritis. However, complicated pyelonephritis requires inpatient treatment with IV antibiotics.

Signs and symptoms that warrant urgent referral also include (Bent et al., 2002; Bremnor & Sadovsky, 2002) the following:

- Patient is unable to provide a clean-catch specimen
- STD is suspected based on history of abnormal discharge or symptoms outside of the genitourinary tract. Of note, presence of a UTI does not rule out a concomitant STD.
- Suspected kidney stones based on hematuria and localized flank pain (usually unilateral)
- Patients with vomiting who cannot tolerate oral fluids
- Pregnant women with suspected pyelonephritis

MAKING THE DIAGNOSIS AND DIFFERENTIAL DIAGNOSES

Diagnostic Testing: Urine Dipstick

The urine dipstick test is a simple way for a convenient care clinic to test urine to screen for a UTI. Some common UTI-causing pathogens produce nitrates as a by-product and white blood cells responding to an infection produce leukocyte esterase.

- *Leukocyte esterase test*: This test is 75% to 96% sensitive and 94% to 98% specific for identifying pyuria. Pyuria may also be seen with a bacterial infection that is not a UTI, such as chlamydial, gonorrheal, or herpetic urethritis.
- *Nitrates*: The test is 22% sensitive and 94% to 100% specific for presence of *Enterobacteriaceae* but lacks adequate sensitivity for the detection of other organisms; thus, a negative result does not rule out a UTI.
- *Hematuria*: This is common in UTI, but in the absence of evidence of infection, referral is warranted to rule out kidney stones or cancer of the urinary tract (Mehnert-Kay, 2005).

Note: A negative or inconclusive dipstick result should not rule out the diagnosis of a UTI when suspicion of infection is highly based on clinical findings. Patients who have taken over-the-counter phenazopyridine may have skewed dipstick results; a decision to refer them for urine microscopy should be based on clinical judgment.

Diagnostic Testing: Urine Culture

The uropathogens responsible for uncomplicated UTI typically respond to empiric therapy, and thus, urine cultures are not generally necessary. However, cultures are indicated for the following:

- Risk factor(s) for complicated UTI, especially pregnancy
- Suspected pyelonephritis
- Negative or inconclusive dipstick when UTI symptoms are otherwise present
- Failure to respond to initial therapy
- All men

A colony-forming unit (CFU) count of $\geq 10^5$/mL has been the standard definition of a positive culture. However, a CFU count of equal to or greater than 10^2/mL may indicate infection, especially if symptoms are present. Antibiotic therapy should be targeted to the sensitivities of the organism (Mehnert-Kay, 2005).

Be sure to obtain a pregnancy test if there is a possibility of pregnancy.

Infectious Differential Diagnosis of Dysuria in Females

Vaginitis: Symptoms may include vaginal discharge and/or odor, vaginal itch, or dyspareunia.

Cervicitis: Symptoms may include abnormal vaginal bleeding and/or discharge, painful sexual intercourse, pain in the vagina, or pressure in the pelvis.

Pelvic inflammatory disease: Chief complaints are fever and abdominal or pelvic pain (Bent et al., 2005; Bremnor & Sadovsky, 2002).

Infectious Differential Diagnosis of Dysuria in Males

Urethritis: Dysuria, with or without discharge, is the typical chief complaint with urethritis, which is much more common in males than UTI. Indications may include a recent new sexual partner and the absence of hematuria. When herpes simplex causes urethritis, symptoms and signs include painful genital ulcers, fever, tender local inguinal lymphadenopathy, and headache.

Acute bacterial prostatitis: Symptoms may include fever, chills, malaise, myalgia, dysuria, cloudy urine, urinary dribbling, or hesitancy.

Chronic prostatitis: Symptoms may include frequency, dysuria, urgency, perineal discomfort, discomfort during ejaculation, deep pelvic pain, or pain radiating to the back. Consider this diagnosis in men with a history of recurrent UTIs in the absence of risk factors such as bladder catheterization.

Acute epididymitis: Symptoms and signs may include dysuria, frequency, urgency, pain in one testicle, high fever, or rigors.

Balanitis and balanoposthitis: Males may develop a nonspecific bacterial infection of the distal penis with involvement of the glans penis (balanitis), or, if uncircumcised, both the glans and the prepuce (balanoposthitis). Symptoms may include penile discharge, pain or difficulty retracting the foreskin, impotence, difficulty urinating or controlling urine stream, tenderness and erythema of the glans penis, or itching (Bremnor & Sadovsky, 2002; Brusch, 2000).

Noninfectious Differential Diagnosis of Dysuria

Irritants: Potential irritants include detergents, fabric softeners, perfumed soaps, and bubble baths. Women may occasionally experience dysuria as a reaction to irritants inserted in the vagina (contraceptive gels, condom, tampons, etc.). Patient history should reveal whether symptoms coincided with introduction of a possible irritant.

Trauma: In both older children and adolescents, normal self-exploratory sexual play, masturbation, voluntary sexual activity, or sexual abuse may be the source of the trauma and urethral irritation. Physical examination is generally unremarkable.

Labial adhesions: These adhesions occur relatively often in young girls. Although they are most frequently asymptomatic, microtears may occasionally cause dysuria.

Urinary stones: Passage of stones may be associated with complaint of dysuria, but flank pain and hematuria are more common.

Urethral strictures: These may present with signs of obstruction such as urinary retention.

Behçet's syndrome: A rare multisystem disease characterized by recurrent oral ulcerations, ocular panuveitis, vasculitis, and, less commonly, genital ulcerations that may produce dysuria.

Atrophic vaginitis: Postmenopausal, estrogen-deficient women can develop dysuria caused by desiccation of the urethral and vaginal mucosa.

Interstitial cystitis: This is a disorder of unknown etiology that occurs predominantly in younger women and is characterized by urgency and frequent voiding of small amounts of urine, often with dysuria or pain but without the evidence of UTI on urinalysis.

Dysfunctional elimination: This is an abnormal pattern of elimination of unknown cause, characterized by both urine and stool incontinence, occurring in previously toilet-trained children without anatomic or neurologic abnormalities. Symptoms may mimic those of a UTI, but it does not usually present acutely (Bent et al., 2002; Bremnor & Sadovsky, 2002; Gupta et al., 2011; Palazzi & Campbell, 2012).

TREATMENT: FIRST LINE, SECOND LINE, AND SUPPORTIVE

In an adult female with uncomplicated UTI, short-course antibiotic therapy is appropriate because of better patient compliance, lower cost, and fewer adverse events. Appropriate first-line drugs include Macrobid, TMP-SFX, or Keflex. If the patient is allergic to sulfa or taking warfarin, then appropriate choices are trimethoprim 100 mg twice daily for 3 days or nitrofurantoin 100 mg twice daily for 5 days. Ciprofloxacin 250 mg twice daily for 3 days is an appropriate second-line choice and is particularly appropriate following recent hospitalization because of the potential for fluoroquinolone or TMP-SMX resistance (American College of Obstetricians and Gynecologists, 2008; Gilbert, Moellering, Eliopoulous, Chambers, & Saag, 2011; Gupta et al., 2011).

Treatment of Complicated UTI

In adult females (Hooton, 2012):

- Ciprofloxacin 500 mg twice daily for 7 to 14 days; levofloxacin 750 mg once daily for 7 to 14 days

In adult males (<50 years: treat for 7 days; ≥50 years: treat for 14 days) (Brusch, 2011):

- TMP-SMX DS twice daily; ciprofloxacin 500 mg twice daily; levofloxacin 250 mg twice daily

Pediatrics (18 months to 17 years) (Palazzi & Campbell, 2012; White, 2011; Zorc, Kiddoo, & Shaw, 2005):

- First line: TMP-SMX 8 mg/kg/d (based on TMP component) twice daily for 10 days (maximum daily dose 320 mg) or cefixime 8 mg/kg twice daily for day 1, then once daily for days 2 to 7 (maximum daily dose 400 mg)
- Second line: cephalexin 50 mg/kg/d once daily for 7 days (maximum daily dose 4,000 mg) or nitrofurantoin 5 to 7 mg/kg/d once daily for 7 days (maximum daily dose 400 mg)

In women who are pregnant (Delzell & Lefevre 2000; Hooton 2012):

- Nitrofurantoin 100 mg twice daily for 5 to 10 days; cephalexin 500 mg twice daily for 7 to 10 days; or amoxicillin-clavulanate 500/125 mg twice daily for 7 to 10 days

- For pain control, acetaminophen and ibuprofen are appropriate, and phenazopyridine 200 mg three times a day for 2 days can be offered to adults 18 years and older with severe dysuria. Adjunctive therapies for dysuria include increased hydration and drinking sugar-free cranberry juice.

RECOMMENDED DISPOSITION AND PATIENT EDUCATION

In addition to the red flags mentioned earlier, follow up with a primary care physician or specialist is indicated for any other abnormal dipstick findings (e.g., ketones or glucose) or for any patient who appears to need further follow-up based on clinical judgment (ICSI, 2006).

Patients should also be given the following take-home points (Brusch, 2011):

- Take the full course of antibiotics as directed. Do not stop taking them just because symptoms improve.
- Drink plenty of water each day
- Avoid carbonated, caffeinated, or alcoholic beverages
- Urinate often, in particular right after sexual intercourse
- Avoid tampons and change sanitary pads often
- Avoid douches, bubble baths, feminine hygiene sprays, and spermicides

- After going to the bathroom, wipe from front to back
- Contact a doctor if symptoms do not improve or if they improve but then return

Patients should be educated to seek immediate medical care if they experience any of the following symptoms or signs (Bent et al., 2002; Bremnor & Sadovsky, 2002):

- Fever, chills, nausea, or vomiting get worse or appear for the first time
- New pain in the back just below the rib cage
- New blood or pus in the urine
- Problems with the antibiotic medicine

Symptoms should have resolved by 48 to 72 hours after the initiation of treatment. If symptoms persist, the patient should be referred for imaging to evaluate for obstructions, investigate alternative diagnoses, and obtain urine culture sensitivities.

Case Resolution: Because the patient had had pyelonephritis within the past year, a urine culture was ordered, and she was given a 7-day course of ciprofloxacin 500 mg twice daily. She was also given patient education, and instructions to go to the ER if she developed any red flag symptoms or signs.

Culture results showed growth of 100,000 colonies of *E. coli*, susceptible to the ciprofloxacin. The patient was notified of the culture results via phone, and she noted improvement in symptoms. She was instructed to finish her entire course of medicine and to follow up with her primary care provider if her symptoms returned or worsened.

SPECIAL CONSIDERATIONS

Pregnancy

Approximately 1% to 2% of pregnant women will develop cystitis; thus, pregnancy tests should be considered in all patients of child-bearing age who present with urinary complaints. Pregnant women should have the same evaluation as those who are not pregnant, but their cases should be treated as complicated UTIs. All pregnant women with a UTI should receive a urine culture and treatment for 3 to 10 days, and fluoroquinolones should be avoided. Pregnant women with pyelonephritis should be hospitalized with IV antibiotics because of the higher risk of complications.

Men

Because of the lower probability of UTI in men, all cases in men should be treated as complicated infections. Thus, urine cultures and a longer course of therapy are mandatory in order to eradicate possible infections of the prostate.

Because nitrofurantoin and β-lactams do not achieve high tissue concentrations in the prostate, they should be avoided. The optimal duration of therapy in men is 7 to 14 days.

Recurrent Infections

Infections are considered recurrent if there are more than two in 6 months or more than three in 1 year. Most repeat infections are actually reinfections; however, relapse due to unresolved infections is possible. CCCs have the responsibility to identify and treat relapse or reinfection and to keep referrals to outside specialists to a minimum. In general, if the second infection occurs less than 2 weeks from the completion of treatment for the first infection, it should be considered recurrent; if it occurs more than 2 weeks later, it should be considered a reinfection. Patients with relapse or reinfection should have cultures ordered and the UTI treated. They should also be referred to a PCP or a specialist, because they may benefit from imaging studies or prophylactic antibiotics.

Pyelonephritis

Pyelonephritis may be beyond the scope of many CCCs' services. Where it is within the clinic's scope, outpatient treatment is an option when the case is mild, and the patient is stable and can tolerate oral fluids. Fluoroquinolones are the only antibiotics recommended for outpatient treatment of acute uncomplicated infections, and these cases require close follow-up as well.

8

Rashes

LORI CREWS AND BRIAN ZELICKSON

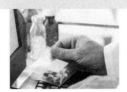

Diagnosing a skin rash is most often accomplished without the use of any special tools other than a good understanding of cutaneous morphology. Many eruptions have several different presentations, whether from different stages of evolution or simply the vast presentations of a single disorder. The good news is that it is not hard to learn the most common patterns of most skin eruptions seen in the convenient care setting. The treatment for these conditions is often straightforward; however, it is important to remember that no treatment should be prescribed without a diagnosis. As tempting as it may be to prescribe topical steroids as a therapeutic trial, this could actually make some diseases worse or create others (Habif, 2004).

This chapter discusses the descriptive vocabulary of a skin eruption so that a correct diagnosis can be made, and other practitioners can understand what you are seeing. It then goes through the most common eruptions seen in convenient care clinics (CCCs).

A thorough history and description of each rash should be obtained and documented. The description of each rash should include all of the following nomenclature:

1. Lesion type
2. Configuration
3. Texture
4. Distribution
5. Color

These comprise the standardized language for describing the clinical manifestations of skin lesions and eruptions (Table 8.1).

The *configuration* of a lesion or eruption that describes the shape of the lesion or cluster of lesions is described as follows:

Linear lesions are in a straight line.
Annular lesions are rings with central clearing.
Nummular lesions are coin shaped or circular.
Target (or bull's-eye) lesions appear as rings.
Reticulated lesions have a lacy or netlike appearance.
Herpetiform lesions are grouped papules or vesicles.
Zosteriform lesions are clustered in a dermatomal distribution.

The *texture* of the eruption is another useful observation.

Verrucous lesions are irregular, pebbly, or rough surfaced.
Lichenification describes a thickening of the texture, which enhances the normal skin markings or dermatoglyphics.
Induration describes a deeper thickening of the skin.
Xanthoma describes yellow, waxy lesions.

The *location* and *distribution* of lesions or eruption should also be documented. Notice whether the lesions are single or multiple, what body parts are affected, and whether the distribution is localized or generalized, random or

Table 8.1 ■ Lesion Types

LESION TYPE	DESCRIPTION
Macule	Flat lesion <1 cm in diameter
Patch	Flat lesion >1 cm in diameter
Papule	Elevated lesions <0.5 cm in diameter
Plaque	Flat-topped elevated lesion >0.5 cm in diameter
Nodule	Raised rounded lesion >0.5 cm in diameter and depth
Vesicle	Blister filled with clear fluid <0.5 cm in diameter
Bullae	Blister filled with clear fluid >0.5 cm in diameter
Pustule	Vesicle filled with pus
Crust	Dried blood or serum
Scale	Dry flaking stratum corneum that is usually white in color
Wheal	Dermal swelling or edema (like a mosquito bite)
Comedones	Acne lesions—black head and white head
Ulcer	Open sore, loss of the epidermis
Erosion	Loss of upper part of the epidermis or superficial sore

patterned, and symmetrical or asymmetrical. It is also good to indicate whether the lesion or eruption is on sun-exposed or sun-protected skin.

The last main descriptor is the *color* of the condition. This usually ranges from flesh colored to white, purple, silver, blue, brown, black, and many shades of red. It will take some time to master the key descriptive nature of many skin conditions, but the most common conditions will be reasonably easy to learn.

COMMON RASHES SEEN IN THE CONVENIENT CARE SETTING

There are numerous skin eruptions that commonly present in CCCs. This chapter focuses on the top rash diagnoses in the convenient care setting.

Eczema or Dermatitis

Eczema or dermatitis is characterized histologically by an inflammatory infiltrate within the epidermis. Clinically, it is most often seen as a red scaly eruption, which is often pruritic. However, there are many presentations and causes of eczema. We examine the most common of these, including allergic and irritant-contact eczema and atopic and seborrheic dermatitis.

Contact Dermatitis

Contact dermatitis is an eruption that arises from the skin in response to an external substance; this substance may be an allergen or an irritant. In allergic contact dermatitis, the reaction is immune mediated and is found only in individuals who are sensitized to the allergen. With irritant dermatitis, on the contrary, the contacting substance directly causes damage to the skin, leading to an inflammatory response in anyone who is exposed to the irritant. The key to diagnosing a contact dermatitis is the location and distribution of the rash as well as a history of exposure. Duration of the rash is also important—the clinical appearance of the eczema can be altered by how long it has been present.

Allergic Contact Dermatitis

To develop an allergic contact dermatitis, one has to have an established sensitivity to that allergen. It usually takes 10 to 14 days to develop a sensitivity reaction after first exposure. Common allergens for contact dermatitis include the plant-based urushiol (found in poison ivy, oak, and sumac), metals such as nickel, fragrances, and topical antibiotics such as neomycin and Bacitracin (see Figure 8.1). Contact dermatitis caused by allergens depends on the person's exposure and genetic makeup. The presentation of contact dermatitis most commonly appears as erythema or edema, with vesicles or

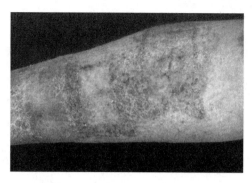

Figure 8.1 ■ Allergic contact dermatitis—poison oak.
(© Wellcome Images/Custom Medical Stock Photo)

papules in a particular linear or streaking configuration on exposed skin such as the hands, legs, or face (Habif, Campbell, Chapman, Dinulos, & Zug, 2006). This configuration is due to direct contact with the allergen. With rhus dermatitis, the eruption is usually in linear or angulated streaks along the areas of contact with the plant. Nickel dermatitis will show up in the areas of contact with jewelry such as the neckline, wrist, or ring finger. The eruption may often spread and grow in intensity for 1 to 2 weeks after contact. However, once the affected area is washed with soap and water, the allergen will no longer transmit the reaction. This is often misunderstood, because the eruption may continue to spread for several days after contact. The chief complaint is often intense pruritus. The intensity of the inflammation increases with the degree of sensitivity, the number of exposures, and the concentration of the antigen.

Treatment of acute allergic contact dermatitis depends on the extent and intensity of the reaction. For acute contact dermatitis, prevention is key, and if there is exposure, it should be followed with copious gentle washing (up to 30 minutes) immediately after exposure. For symptomatic relief of acute dermatitis, cool compresses, calamine lotion, and oatmeal baths can be helpful. Other topical agents such as Burow's solution or Zanfel can relieve symptoms (Prok & McGovern, 2012). Acute dermatitis will also benefit from high-potency topical steroids (clobetasol propionate 0.05% cream) when the dermatitis is severe; however, these agents should not be used on the face, genitals, or intertriginous areas (Weston & Howe, 2011). Cases of severe extensive acute contact dermatitis, especially those involving the face, will benefit from oral steroids. Because of the prolonged immune response, oral prednisone should be used in a 14- to 21-day taper. Most of these patients will have complete resolution of symptoms; however, if the condition worsens or fails to improve, the patient should be reexamined for rebounding or a superinfection. Treatment for either subacute or chronic allergic contact dermatitis is similar and features the use of topical steroids for limited-distribution rashes. Oral steroids will be needed for more extensive areas of contact dermatitis or more severe cases. A medrol dose pack or a 1- to 2-week tapering dose is usually sufficient (Weston & Howe, 2011).

Antihistamines may help both types of dermatitis, particularly first-generation ones because of their sedating effects.

Irritant-Contact Dermatitis

Irritant-contact dermatitis a non-immune-mediated response that results in a specific configuration when an external chemical causes direct irritation of the skin. Irritants may be as weak as mild hand soap or as aggressive as industrial chemicals. The presentation can vary from mild itching and erythema to dry skin with fissuring to blisters and open erosions. The reaction can appear after a single exposure or a series of exposures to the agent. Once the offending irritant is avoided, the rash does not spread. Again, a history of exposure is key to the diagnosis.

Treatment of irritant dermatitis is removal and avoidance of the offending agent. With blistering or weeping eruptions, wet compresses may be effective to heal the skin. The cool compresses should be used 15 to 30 minutes several times a day until the severe itching is controlled. Topical steroids will help suppress erythema and itching in the acute phase. However, unless avoidance is maintained in the future, the reaction will reoccur (Habif, 2004).

Atopic Dermatitis

Atopic dermatitis is a genetic immune condition that can be seen in all ages; there are usually no single causative agents. It is called the itch that rashes. Often the patient will describe that an itch appeared first; that when the itch was rubbed or scratched, the area continued to itch more; and that with this cycle of itching and scratching, the rash appeared (see Figure 8.2). The eruption most often occurs in winter or dry seasons. The general distribution is symmetrical and in the antecubital and popliteal fossa in children and adults but can be on the face and buttocks in infants. Atopic dermatitis is often accompanied by a personal or family history of hay fever and/or asthma. Some contact irritants or allergens can aggravate atopic dermatitis, including wool clothing, fragrances (such as those in laundry detergents or fabric softeners), and preservatives.

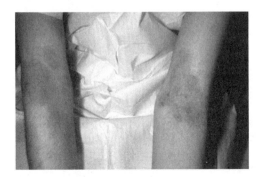

Figure 8.2 ▪ Atopic dermatitis often appears more erythematous, as can be seen in this image.
(© Custom Medical Stock Photo)

Treatment includes avoiding any offending agents, hydrating the skin, topical anti-inflammatory medication, and possible antihistamines or oral prednisone if the itching is severe and the rash extensive. Hydrating the skin is very important and quite easy. The best way is to take a warm—not hot—shower or bath, lightly towel off to leave some moisture on the skin, and apply a heavy, fragrance-free cream to help seal in the moisture. Bath oil can also be used in the bath or put in a spray bottle and sprayed on after a shower. A mid-potency topical corticosteroid can be applied to the area twice per day for 2 to 4 weeks. A low-potency topical corticosteroid should be used only for a short time in the groin and flexural areas to avoid skin atrophy. If there is an associated infection, it should be treated with topical and/or oral antibiotics and antiseptic moist compresses. A very easy antiseptic compress is made by mixing 1 ounce of white vinegar with 1 quart of warm tap water and moistening a clean cotton towel with the mixture; compress the area for 10 to 20 minutes two to three times per day.

Seborrheic Dermatitis

Commonly referred to as dandruff, seborrheic dermatitis can occur at all ages but appears most commonly in adults. It involves the development of scaly red patches in areas of sebaceous glands, and there is mild to moderate pruritus as well. Seborrheic dermatitis presents as a reddish, scaly eruption in hair-bearing areas such as the scalp, eyebrows, and mid-chest in men; a classic presentation is dandruff of the scalp. It can also affect the mid-face and postauricular area or external auditory canals. The condition is thought to be the result of an inflammatory reaction to a commensal organism that lives in our skin, and it tends to be worse during the winter months. The best therapy includes the use of medicated shampoos containing zinc pyrithione, selenium, tar, salicylic acid, selenium sulfide, and/or ketoconazole. The two most common dandruff shampoos are selenium sulfide 2.5% and ketoconazole 2%, and it is best to leave the shampoo in place for a few minutes before washing it off. In nonscalp seborrheic dermatitis, topical steroid creams, nonsteroidal anti-inflammatory creams, and ketoconazole cream are the most effective.

Urticaria (Hives)

Another common skin disorder, hives are classified as acute or chronic—they have the same presentation, appearing as circular lesions or erythema with a central area of pallor (see Figure 8.3).

In acute urticaria, the individual lesions usually last 1 to 3 days, and the condition often resolves in 1 to 3 weeks; it can, however, last several months. The cause of the condition is identified in fewer than 20% of cases (Reeves & Maibach, 1998). Some causes include ingestion of certain pharmaceuticals, viruses, bacterial infections, foods or food additives, and latex, to name a few. The lesions develop when mast cells release histamines and vasodilators and other mediators of inflammation in response to an antigen. The lesions present as wheals that are circumscribed, erythematous, edematous papules, and

Figure 8.3 ■ In severe cases of urticaria, lesions can become confluent.
Notice the raised appearance of the hives.
(© Wellcome Images/Custom Medical Stock Photo)

plaque that is usually pruritic. Hives are usually red and erythematous and may be round or oval shaped. The most severe complaint is usually the itch. The wheal can change in size and shape, and new lesions may evolve as others resolve (Habif, 2004). Hives are occasionally associated with angioedema. When evaluating patients, it is important to inquire about systemic illness, including difficulty breathing, tightness of the throat, lightheadedness, or other signs of anaphylaxis.

Treating hives includes trying to identify the offending agent and eliminating it and treating the symptoms with oral antihistamines and topical anti-inflammatory medications. First-line drugs should be the second-generation H1 antihistamines, as they are minimally sedating and have fewer side effects. These drugs include cetirizine, loratadine, and fexofenadine. First-generation H1 antihistamines such as diphenhydramine and hydroxyzine can be used, but their side-effect profile of sedation and other cognitive affects must be considered. A brief course of glucocorticoids (40–60 mg every day for 5 days) can be used in addition to antihistamines for persistent or severe symptoms. Patients suspected of having an anaphylactic reaction should be emergently referred, and patients with suspected allergic etiologies to a food or medication should be referred nonurgently for allergy testing.

Chronic urticaria, which is found in only 5% of cases, is diagnosed when urticaria lasts longer than 3 months. The precipitators may be similar to those in acute cases and may also include vitamins, laxatives, mints, toothpaste, and nonmedicinal substances, but often the cause cannot be identified (Reeves & Maibich, 1998).

Obtaining a thorough patient history is of utmost importance and includes asking about any medications, vitamins, changes in diet, recent insect stings, illnesses, or emotional stress to which the patient has been exposed. Reassure the patient that in the majority of cases, the cause is never identified. Treatment for both acute and chronic urticaria includes removing the precipitants or triggers if identified, and topical therapy includes cool baths, corticosteroids, and calamine lotion. A complete general medical examination is required for working up chronic urticaria; hence, patients should be referred to their primary physicians

Signs and Symptoms of Anaphylaxis

- Difficulty breathing, feeling like the throat is tightening up
- Syncope or near syncopal events, feeling lightheaded
- Having a feeling of flush or warmth with severe swelling or angioedema
- Wheezing or stridor on examination
- Gastrointestinal (GI) distress, nausea, vomiting, or diarrhea
- Chest pain, chest tightness, palpitations, tachyarrhythmias, low blood pressure
- Anxiety
- Altered mental status or confusion

or dermatologists. Systemic agents include antihistamines, nonsedating, and/or traditional sedating antihistamines at bedtime.

Scabies

Scabies is a highly pruritic eruption that brings patients to the convenient care setting (see Figure 8.4). The human eye is unable to detect the culprit, which is *Sarcoptes scabiei* var. *hominis*, or the human itch mite. This tiny mite burrows in to the top layer

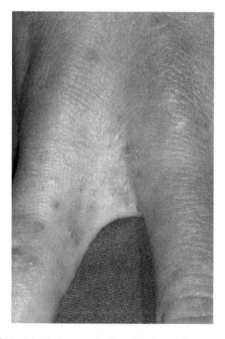

Figure 8.4 ■ Scabies lesions: note the raised, papular nature of the lesion. Notice the marks between the digits, which is a common place to find the reddish lesions. The patient will report an intense itching sensation.
(© Science Photo Library/Custom Medical Stock Photo)

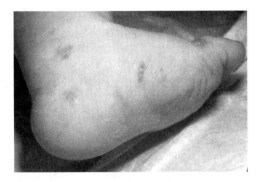

Figure 8.5 ■ Scabies burrow.
(© Custom Medical Stock Photo)

of dead skin and lays eggs (see Figure 8.5). The eggs hatch around day 5, these mites reproduce, and more eggs are added in the top layer of skin. This initial phase can produce a few hundred mites before the human host experiences an eruption or itching. It is in the second phase, 2 or 3 weeks after the initial invasion, that the patient develops an allergic response to the mites. Most often there are less than 2 dozen mites infesting the patient.

The eruption can be extremely itchy and seems to present worse at night. It is usually after the second week of infestation that patients present to the clinic with the complaint of a red, itchy eruption that may be hindering a good night's rest. The most common locations are the wrists, finger webs, and belly button—looking closely, one can often see a tiny linear burrow in these areas. Younger children may present with the eruption covering the entire body. Older children and adults rarely have the presentation of this eruption above the neck or on the palms and soles (Reeves & Maibach, 1998).

At one time, scabies was attributed to poor hygiene. In clinical settings today, the majority of cases seem to appear in patients with adequate hygiene, usually those with contact with a lot of other people, including possibly school-children. Scabies is passed in families, neighborhoods, or areas where inanimate objects such as clothes or towels are shared freely. It can also be spread by intimate personal contact. Scabies is rarely spread without human contact but may occasionally be shed into clothing or bedding; however, because the mite lives less than 24 hours without human contact, this is a rare occurrence.

The good news for the patient is that this is an easily treated disease. A scabicide such as permethrin 5% lotion should be applied to the entire body, from neck to feet. The lotion should be left on overnight and washed off in the morning. Treatment should include application between fingers, umbilicus, genitalia, and body folds. Caution the patient that the pruritus may last 2 or 3 weeks after treatment, as the body will still be reacting to this allergic invasion. As with other cases of allergic dermatitis, an antihistamine may be used to provide the patient comfort. An oral treatment, ivermectin, is also approved for treatment of scabies.

Patients or parents of patients need to be informed of the sources of possible scabies transmission. All family members or those in close personal contact with the patient should be treated at the same time. If there are any pets in the house, they should be checked by a veterinarian as well. All bedclothing, towels, and night clothes should be washed the morning following treatment. If any bedding is difficult to clean, it should be set aside for a couple of days, since the mite cannot live more than 24 hours without human contact.

Impetigo

Impetigo is a common, very contagious, bacterial skin infection commonly found in school-age children (see Figure 8.6). Hot, humid environments and crowded, poor socioeconomic conditions may also increase the risk (Reeves & Maibach, 1998). The eruption or infection will spread from one part of the body to another by scratching. Impetigo is caused by *Staphylococcus aureus* and/or

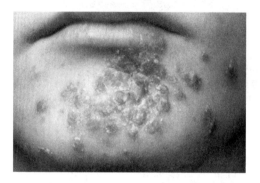

Figure 8.6 ■ Impetigo hallmarked by a crusted lesion, which is often honey colored.
(© Wellcome Images/Custom Medical Stock Photo)

Streptococcus pyogenes. There are two types of impetigo, bullous and nonbullous. Nonbullous impetigo is the most common form and presents as a red area with vesicles that become pustules, which then rupture and create a thick, honey-colored crust. Bullous impetigo consists of vesicles that enlarge to form blisters that persist (see Figure 8.7). Topical therapy should be used in nonbullous impetigo with a limited number of lesions. Treatment of choice is mupirocin 2% ointment or cream three times per day for 10 days. Oral antibiotics should be used when the lesions are bullous or are extensive. First-line choices

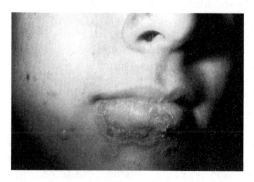

Figure 8.7 ■ Bullous impetigo.
(© Custom Medical Stock Photo)

include cephalexin, dicloxacillin, or clindamycin, and treatment should be for 7 days. Appropriate hand hygiene instructions are essential.

Herpes Simplex (HSV-1)

HSV-1 presents with grouped painful papules or vesicles on the lips and oral mucosa (see Figure 8.8). It may be preceded by a painful or itching prodrome in the area. After initial infection, the virus is reactivated through the trigeminal sensory ganglion. Primary infections usually last longer and are associated with more systemic symptoms. The lesions usually occur on the lips and can be initiated by sun exposure or injury from the dentist. Although clear vesicles are present, they do not ooze and create a honey-colored crust. The eruption can last at least 2 weeks.

Treatment includes antiviral medication starting within 48 hours of presentation of the eruption. Antiviral agents include famciclovir, valacyclovir, and acyclovir. Early treatment leads to shorter duration of illness as well as a diminished infectious stage. Pain medication can be used for comfort. Topical medications such as magic mouthwash or lidocaine are helpful. Duration of therapy is usually 7 to 10 days. For patients with recurrent infections who sense an impending flare (prodrome), it is reasonable to treat with single-day dosing of famciclovir or valacyclovir (Klein, 2012).

Varicella/Herpes Zoster (Shingles)

Caused when the chicken pox virus reactivates after lying dormant in the sensory ganglia of a patient who in the past has had chicken pox. It presents as an extremely painful rash of grouped linear papules and vesicles in a dermatomal

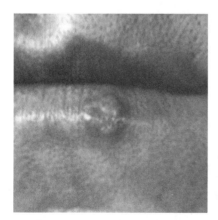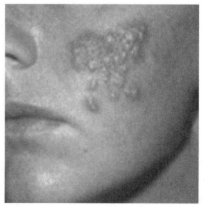

Figure 8.8 ■ Herpes simplex: Oral lesions classically appear on the lip, but can occur in other dermatomal distributions.
(http://medicalpicturesinfo.com/herpes)

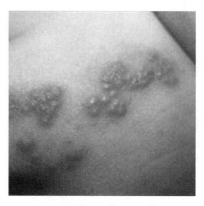

Figure 8.9 ■ The classic vesicular appearance of herpes zoster or shingles.
(http://medicalpicturesinfo.com/herpes-zoster)

distribution (see Figures 8.9 and 8.10). Within 7 to 10 days, the lesions will crust over. The key to making the diagnosis is the finding of vesicles that exist in one to two dermatomal regions. It can be accompanied with a low-grade fever and upper respiratory symptoms and can be very painful or pruritic.

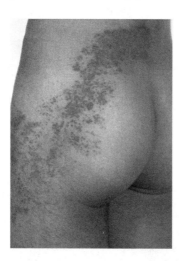

Figure 8.10 ■ Herpes zoster in a dermatomal distribution.
(© Wellcome Image Library/Custom Medical Stock Photo)

The goals of treatment are to diminish pain, decrease duration of the lesions, and prevent postherpetic complications such as neuralgia. Oral antiviral and pain medication should be initiated as early as possible, ideally within 72 hours of clinical presentation. Agents include acyclovir, valacyclovir, and famciclovir. It is important to control the pain, because it can persist beyond the resolution of the eruption and often require opiate medications. The role of steroids in treating zoster is controversial; as of publication of this text, their use is out of favor because of the increased risk of secondary infection.

Cellulitis

Cellulitis is a skin infection that presents as areas of red, warm, painful skin. Occasionally, it can present with drainage of purulent material, which is usually associated with the formation of an abscess. Cellulitis can be diagnosed and treated in the CCC. However, immunosuppressed patients, extensive cellulitis, facial involvement, or systemic involvement (e.g., high fever and low blood pressure) should be emergently referred. Diabetics with lower extremity cellulitis should also be urgently referred. In addition, pain out of proportion to the physical examination should be referred for imaging because of the possibility of necrotizing fasciitis. Beta-hemolytic streptococci and *S. aureus* are the most common offending agents.

Cellulitis should be treated with antibiotics and by keeping the affected extremity elevated. Antibiotic selection will vary depending on local prevalence of methicillin-resistant Staphylococcus aureus (MRSA) strains. First-line antibiotics for treating cellulitis in areas of low MRSA include dicloxacillin, cephalexin, or clindamycin. In areas with high MRSA prevalence, in patients with a history of MRSA or who fail first-line treatment, or in cases of recurrence, drugs of choice include oral clindamycin, tetracycline, and trimethoprim-sulfamethoxazole. Treatment should be for 7 to 10 days. The area of redness should be demarcated with a pen or marker and patients instructed to seek medical attention if the infection spreads outside of the marked area. Patients should have follow-up within 1 to 2 days.

Burn

Occasionally, minor burns will present to the CCC. The primary role for the clinician is to distinguish between minor and more severe burns that require a higher level of care. In evaluating burns, first define the thickness of the burn (or the depth), and then describe the size or the extent of the burn. With depth, one should distinguish superficial from partial thickness or full thickness burns. Superficial burns (first degree) represent damage to the epidermal layer; they will be red and painful without blisters and will blanch white with pressure. Partial thickness burns (second degree) represent damage to the epithelial and partial damage to the dermal level. They will blister and be painful and will also blanch with pressure, but will not have damaged the hair follicles or deeper structures. In general, first-degree and minor second-degree burns can easily be managed on an outpatient basis and will heal with minimal to no scarring.

Full or partial thickness burns should be referred to a specialist because of the potential for scarring. After it is determined whether it is a first- or second-degree burn, the size of the burn should be documented as a percentage of total body surface area; an easy guide is to use the palm of your hand to represent 5% of the body. In general, more extensive burns (i.e., second-degree burns greater than 10% in adults or 5% in pediatrics), as well as burns of the face or the genital region, may require referral (see Figure 8.11). Other burns that require close follow-up or referral are circumferential second-degree burns on the hands or on the feet. In general, first-degree burns are appropriate to

---

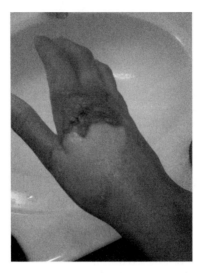

Figure 8.11 ■ Although this burn looks serious, the fact that it is still painful to the touch classifies it as a second-degree or partial thickness burn. Burns of the hand should be referred to a burn center.
(http://ookaboo.com/o/pictures/picture/12515542/ Seconddegree_burn_caused_by_contact_with)

care for in the CCC as they are most commonly caused by sunburns (see Figure 8.12). Treatment involves cleaning any wounds with soap and water. Blisters that are ruptured should be removed, but intact blisters can remain intact. Patients will require pain management with nonsteroidal anti-inflamatory drugs (NSAIDs) or acetaminophen with opioids as needed. Topical coverage with Bacitracin can help with healing and prevent superinfection. Silver

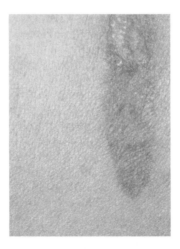

Figure 8.12 ■ Sunburn is a first-degree burn with a small area of second-degree burn as manifested by the blisters.
(© A. Wilson/Custom Medical Stock Photo)

sulfadiazine, once popular in treatment of burns, is thought to slow healing and is best avoided. Tetanus prophylaxis should be offered if needed. For comfort, a dressing should be applied, which should include a base layer of a nonadherent dressing.

Tinea (Fungal Infections)

Tinea are superficial inflammatory or noninflammatory infections caused by dermatophytes and also commonly seen in the CCC. The most common of these dermatophytes are *Trichophyton, Microsporum*, and *Epidermophyton*. The organisms invade the stratum corneum and mostly reside in this layer and the upper live epidermis, although occasionally they will invade the cutaneous adnexa and dermis. The infections spread contiguously, often causing an erythematous nummular eruption. Tinea infections can be seen in all ages. Tinea capitis and corporis are most often seen in children and adolescents and often result from close contact with other people or animals with an infection. Extensive tinea infections can also be seen in immunocompromised persons.

There is often scaling seen at the edge of the lesions, which is a natural defense mechanism resulting in shedding of the stratum corneum. It is these nummular lesions with a scaling periphery that have given fungal infections the common term ringworm. Fungal infections are most often found in hot, humid environments. They are described by the area that is infected: Tinea corporis involves the glaborious skin of the body and is most often caused by *Trichophyton rubrum*; tinea capitis involves the scalp and is most often caused by *Trichophyton tonsurans*; and tinea pedis and tinea manuum are infections of the feet and hands, respectively, whereas onychomycosis involves infection of the nails. Most infections are asymptomatic or cause mild itching. If there is significant itching or pain, the patients should be suspected of being immunocompromised. Most often, the eruption consists of mild erythematous macules with fine peripheral scaling, but can be more inflammatory, with edema, vesicles, and/or blisters. Confirmation of the diagnosis can be accomplished with a KOH preparation and/or culture of a skin scraping.

Treatment includes determining and treating the source of the infection such as house pets or farm animals. Most cases of tinea can be treated and controlled with over-the-counter (OTC) antifungal creams including the topical azoles (e.g., econazole, ketoconazole, clotrimazole, miconazole, oxiconazole, sulconazole) or the topical allylamines (e.g., naftifine, terbinafine) twice per day for 2 to 4 weeks. A mild- to medium-potency topical corticosteroid may be used to help with accompanying inflammation. The area should also be kept cool and dry to prevent reinfection. Some tinea infections, especially those involving the toe webs, can be combined bacterial infections and should be treated with both topical antifungal and antibiotic creams. If infections do not clear in 2 to 4 weeks, patients should be referred to a dermatologist. Onychomycosis infections most often need oral antifungals and should be referred to a dermatologist.

CONCLUSION

Knowing the morphology of the dermatologic conditions that commonly present at CCCs is critical for correct diagnosis and management. Patients with abnormal presentations, those who do not respond to therapy, or those with symptoms that are out of the scope of service for the convenient care setting should be referred to a dermatologist.

9

Fever

KILEY BLACK

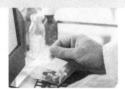

Fever, in children and adults, is a common chief complaint seen in the convenient care clinic (CCC) setting. It is especially prevalent in children, accounting for "approximately one-third of all pediatric outpatient visits in the United States" (Finkelstein, Christiansen, & Platt, 2000, p. 260). This chapter focuses on the assessment and treatment of pediatric fever.

Fever itself is not an illness; rather, it is a normal central nervous system response to endogenous (e.g., leukemia) or exogenous (e.g., bacteria) pyrogens. In other words, fever is a defense mechanism of the body, and it plays an integral part in the overall inflammatory response. Whether a fever is beneficial or harmful remains unclear in medical research literature (Ward, 2012). Potential benefits include reducing the growth of bacteria and viruses by essentially "baking" them and strengthening the overall immune system response; the primary downside is the increased demand fever places on other body systems such as cardiac or pulmonary, which may lead to shock in those systems due to increased cardiac output and oxygen consumption (Mackowiak, 1994).

Case Study: A 3-year-old female is brought to the CCC by her father. She is taken into the exam room at the start of the visit. Her father reports that his daughter has been home with a fever for 2 days, with the most recent reading being 102.0°F using an axillary thermometer. He also says his wife gave the patient a pediatric dose of aceta-minophen about 5 hours ago, but he can't remember the amount.

According to the father, the patient hasn't complained of any other associated symptoms such as a sore throat, cough, ear pain, or dysuria. She has been more "clingy" the past 2 days. Her father reports that the patient is eating, drinking, and urinating normally. Her immunizations are current. She attends day care, and her father thinks there may have been strep going around at the center recently. The patient has not received any antibiotics in the past 3 months, and there are no ill contacts at home. The father is very concerned about his daughter's high fever and states she "needs an antibiotic now." Review of systems is negative except for a history of bilateral ear infections at age 2. Physical examination findings are as follows:

Vital signs: T = 101.9°F orally, pulse = 120, respirations = 22, BP = 80 systolic, pulse oximetry = 98% RA

General: No acute distress. Well developed and well nourished. Cooperative with examination. Smiles at practitioner.

HEENT:

Head—normocephalic, atraumatic; bilateral maxillary and frontal sinuses non-tender to palpation

Eyes—PERRLA, EOMI, conjunctiva non-injected bilaterally

Ears—Bilateral external canals are free of edema, erythema, and exudate; right TM is pearly gray, intact, and without erythema or edema; left TM is mildly erythematous but intact and without edema

Nose—pink and moist; no discharge

Mouth/Throat—moist oral membranes; mild pharyngeal erythema; tonsils are without erythema or exudate

Respiratory: Clear to auscultation bilaterally; no use of accessory muscles, no nose flaring

Cardiovascular: RRR, S1, and S2 present; no murmur, gallop, or rub appreciated

Abdomen: bowel sounds present in all four quadrants, no pain with palpation

Integumentary: good skin turgor, no rashes

Lymph: no lymphadenopathy

A rapid strep test is negative; a throat culture is sent to an outside laboratory

Terminology used in clinical practice to describe fever is perplexing. Despite popular belief, there is no specific "normal body temperature"; core body temperature follows a circadian rhythm and can be affected by many factors such as age, exercise, and menstrual cycle. Specific terms such as "fever of unknown origin" and "fever without source" have been used in the literature with varying definitions. For the purpose of this chapter, the generic terms "fever" and "fever with concern" will be used with specified parameters (Ward, 2012) (see Table 9.1). A commonly defined cutoff for referral from a CCC to a tertiary care facility is 103.0 to 104.0°F (39.4°–40.0°C).

Table 9.1 ■ Parameters for Fever With Concern

AGE	METHOD	FEVER	FEVER OF CONCERN
0–3 months*	Rectal		100.4–100.7°F (≥38.0–38.2°C)
3–36 months*	Rectal	100.4–102.2°F (≥38.0–39.0°C)	≥102.2°F (≥39.0°C)
Older children/ adults	Oral	100.0°–103.1°F (≥37.8–39.4°C)	≥103.1°F (≥39.5°C)

*Pediatric patients not seen at CCCs until 18 to 24 months.

OVERALL APPROACH

Fever can be an anxiety-provoking situation for not only parents but health care professionals as well. "Fever phobia" is a term coined by B. D. Schmitt (1980) when he found that "the great concern of parents about fever is not justified" (p. 176). Medical professionals may contribute to this phobia, particularly when there is not a clear diagnosis. May and Bauchner (1992) note that "clinical experience suggests that pediatricians may impart mixed messages to patients about the dangers of fever" (p. 851). An overall clinical approach to the child with fever provides a systemic way to guide the clinician through the interaction and helps to alleviate anxiety for both parties.

Shah (2012) promotes a three-phase approach to the fever patient, with specific instructions for each phase. Phase 1, shown in Table 9.2, is particular to the CCC setting; phases 2 and 3 require invasive testing and are out of the scope of a CCC.

Assessment

In otherwise healthy children, most fevers are self-limiting and benign (Ward, 2012). In fact, 40% to 60% of fevers in children resolve without identification of a specific cause (Shah, 2012). Luszczak (2001) acknowledged that "the overwhelming majority of non-toxic but febrile children have a viral infection" (p. 1219).

However, there are several factors that indicate an increased risk for bacteremia or sepsis in children. These include being under the age of 2 months, in an immunocompromised state, being un- or under-vaccinated, and hyperthermia (core temp >40.5°C or 105°F). Given these risk factors, the National Institute of Health and Clinical Excellence guidelines suggest performing a clinical assessment in three stages for children younger than 5 years (Richardson & Lakhanpaul, 2007, p. 1163):

1. Check for any life-threatening symptoms (airway, breathing, circulation, and disability). If there are any, refer immediately for emergency medical care.
2. Assess the risk of serious illness using the Traffic Light System (Table 9.3)
3. Attempt to identify a focus of infection or features of specific serious conditions

Table 9.2 ■ Approach to Fever in the Convenient Care Setting

Phase 1 Assessment	• Document fever
	• Perform a thorough history and physical examination
	• Determine whether constitutional symptoms suggest an underlying disease process
	• Develop differential diagnosis list
	• Begin initial noninvasive lab tests as indicated by evaluation

Table 9.3 ■ The Traffic Light System for Risk Assessment

CATEGORY	LOW RISK	MEDIUM RISK	HIGH RISK
Skin color	• Normal color of skin, lips, and tongue	• Pallor reported by caregiver or noted by practitioner	• Pale, mottled, ashen, or blue
Activity	• Responds normally to social cues • Is content or smiles • Stays awake or awakens quickly • Strong normal cry or not crying	• Doesn't respond normally to social cues • Wakes only with prolonged stimulation • Decreased activity • No smiling	• No response to social overtures • Unrousable or does not stay awake if roused • Weak, high-pitched, or continuous cry
Respiration	• Normal	• Nasal flaring • Tachypnea • Oxygen saturation • Crackles on auscultation	• Grunting • Tachypnea • Moderate to severe chest retractions
Hydration	• Normal skin and eyes • Moist mucus membranes	• Dry mucus membranes • Poor feeding • Capillary refill ≥3 s • Reduced urine output	• Reduced skin turgor
Other	• No yellow or red features	• Swelling of a limb or joint • Non–weight bearing or not using an extremity	• Nonblanching rash • Bulging fontanelle • Neck stiffness • Status epilepticus • Focal neurological signs • Focal seizures • Bile-stained vomiting

Source: Richardson and Lakhanpaul (2007).

History of Present Illness/Review of Systems

A complete and thorough history is warranted when evaluating a patient with a fever, particularly if he or she appears to be asymptomatic. Important history questions to ask include the following (Graneto, 2011):

- Immunization history (recent vaccinations and incomplete series)
- History of recent exposure to sick contacts at daycare, school, or home; daycare attendance has been identified as a risk factor for otitis media (Luszczak, 2001)
- Recent travel history

- History of prematurity, immunocompromised status, or recent hospitalization (including ICU stay)
- Recent change in eating and/or behavioral patterns such as irritability, lethargy, or apnea
- Received antibiotic therapy within past 3 to 6 months
- History of neglect or abuse (may be difficult to assess in HPI but watch for physical examination findings)

In addition, obtaining a detailed fever history is essential. Palazzi (2012) recommends the following:

- What was the duration and height of the fever?
- How was the fever assessed (e.g., by touch, forehead strip, or thermometer)?
- Was the fever confirmed by someone other than the parent or caregiver? Studies have shown that parental subjective fever assessment (e.g., feeling the forehead) is a reliable indicator of a fever having been present (Graneto, 2011).
- Are there any specific circumstances that preceded the fever?
- If antipyretics were given, what was the dose, when was it last given, and how quickly did the fever respond to the drugs?
- What has been the predominant fever pattern (remittent, intermittent, sustained, or relapsing)?

Physical Examination

The goal of the physical examination is to identify a source or reason for the fever, with specific attention to potential serious infections such as meningitis. Table 9.4 shows the clinical features of specific severe diseases in conjunction with fever. Several examination findings, as identified by Graneto (2011), can be obtained by observing the child's interaction with the parent and the practitioner. Watch for the following:

- If patient is crying, what is the quality of the cry? Is it abnormal, high-pitched, or weak in effort? Are tears being produced while the child is crying?
- Is the child fearful of the practitioner? Beyond infancy, healthy young children should have a reasonable fear of strangers. The child who lies on the examination bed without much interaction or response to examination may be more likely to have a serious illness.
- What is the skin color? Are there areas of cyanosis or jaundice? Are there any rashes present? For example, petechiae have been associated with bacteremia, viral, and rickettsial infections, and infectious endocarditis (Palazzi, 2012).
- What is the degree of hydration? Is there moisture on the oral mucosa, lips, or tongue?
- What is the response to social overtures? A social smile in younger children is one of the better predictors of healthy children.

Table 9.4 ■ Clinical Symptoms of Specific Serious Infections in Conjunction With Fever

Kawasaki disease	*Urinary tract infection*
Fever for more than 5 days and at least four of the following:	• Vomiting
• Bilateral conjunctival injection	• Poor feeding
• Change in mucus membranes	• Lethargy
• Change in the extremities	• Irritability
• Polymorphous rash	• Abdominal pain or tenderness
• Cervical lymphadenopathy	• Urinary frequency or urgency
	• Offensive urine or hematuria
Herpes simplex encephalitis	*Septic arthritis or osteomyelitis*
• Focal neurological signs	• Swelling of limb or joint
• Focal seizures	• Not using extremity
• Decreased level of consciousness	• Non-weight bearing
Meningococcal disease	*Meningitis*
Nonblanching rash with one or more of the following:	• Neck stiffness
• Child looks ill	• Bulging fontanelle
• Lesions larger than 2 mm in diameter (purpura)	• Decreased level of consciousness
• A capillary refill time of ≥3 seconds	• Convulsive status epilepticus
• Neck stiffness	

Pneumonia
- Cyanosis
- Tachypnea: respiratory rate > 40/min if age > 12 months
- Nasal flaring
- Chest indrawing
- Crackles on auscultation
- Oxygen saturation 95%

A thorough physical examination should be performed with special attention paid to skin; ear, nose, and throat; lung; heart; and neurological systems. Several pearls in clinical practice include checking capillary refill time, performing a thorough respiratory system examination, and carefully auscultating the heart sounds.

- Capillary refill time is generally thought to be the quickest early assessment of hypoperfusion. A delay in time (≥3 seconds) indicates shunting of the blood from the capillary beds in the skin and relates to increased systemic vascular resistance (SVR). An increase in SVR is thought to occur in the course of pediatric hypovolemia.
- The presence of dyspnea, tachypnea, grunting, flaring, and retractions suggests possible serious illness and requires further exploration (e.g., chest x-ray).
- Examination of the chest may reveal findings consistent with pneumonia. The presence of a cardiac murmur, especially new onset, may suggest infective endocarditis.

DIAGNOSIS

Selecting a diagnosis involves clinical judgment and decision making. This step may provoke trepidation in the practitioner, because conventional wisdom requires specific information in order to create a treatment plan. Starting with a differential diagnosis list may make the process less intimidating.

Differential Diagnosis

Once the examination has been completed, developing a list of differential diagnoses is quite helpful in determining the next course of action. As one can imagine, the differential diagnosis for fever is exhaustive and includes both infectious and noninfectious options. Table 9.5 lists common infectious causes of fever, less common infectious causes, and noninfectious causes.

Table 9.5 ■ Common Causes of Fever

COMMON INFECTIOUS CAUSES	LESS COMMON INFECTIOUS CAUSES	NONINFECTIOUS CAUSES
Otitis media	Tuberculosis	Collagen vascular disease (juvenile rheumatoid arthritis, lupus)
Sinusitis	Infectious mononucleosis	Malignancy
Pharyngitis	Lyme disease	Kawasaki syndrome
Upper respiratory illness	Rickettsial disease	Inflammatory bowel disease
Urinary tract infection	Malaria	Drug fever
Pneumonia	Bacterial or viral meningitis	Factitious fever or Munchausen syndrome by proxy
Peritonsillar abscess	Dental or periodontal abscess	Centrally mediated fever
Bone or joint infection	Acute rheumatic fever	
Enteric infection (e.g., *Salmonella*)	HIV	
Cat-scratch disease	Toxoplasmosis	
Influenza	Endemic fungi	
Bronchiolitis (RSV)	Sepsis/bacteremia	

Source: Adapted from Shah (2012).

Diagnostic Testing

Several sources recommend obtaining a complete blood count, blood and urine culture, and chest x-ray on children with high fevers; these tests (with the exception of the urine culture) are typically not available in the convenient care setting. However, the inability to perform a chest x-ray or blood work should not result in an automatic referral to a higher level of service. Available to the retail-based clinician are several Clinical Laboratory Improvement Act–waived point-of-care (POC) tests that offer useful diagnostic information. Several POC tests that may help to determine a diagnosis are the following:

- Rapid strep/throat culture
- Urine analysis/urine culture
- Influenza test
- Mononucleosis test
- TB Mantoux test

It is not a standard of care to perform every test on a patient in the hopes of identifying a source of the fever. Rather, the decision to run specific POC tests should be made in conjunction with all other information collected from the patient and taking into account the prevalence of very common infections seen in children. Table 9.6A through Table 9.6C show the prevalence of certain diagnoses.

Case Study Diagnosis: Reflecting back to the clinical scenario, the 3-year-old most likely has a viral illness that she may have been exposed to in day care. Because the clinician is unable to identify the virus causing the illness, the diagnosis is simply fever, unspecified.

Table 9.6A ■ UTI

DEMOGRAPHIC GROUP	PREVALENCE OR PRETEST PROBABILITY (95% CI)
0–24 months	
Girls	7.3%
White girls with temperature ≥39°C	16%
Boys	8.0%
White children	8.0%
Black children	4.7%
<19 years with fever and/or urinary symptoms	7.8%

Source: Shaikh and Hoberman (2012).

Table 9.6B ■ **Otitis Media**

RISK FACTOR	RELATIVE RISK (RR) (95% CI)
Family history	2.63
Day care	2.45
Lack of breastfeeding	Unknown
Tobacco smoke and air pollution	1.66
Pacifier use	1.24
Race and ethnicity	Native Americans, Alaskan and Canadian Eskimos, and indigenous Australian children have increased risk

Source: Klein and Pelton (2012).

Table 9.6C ■ **Pharyngitis**

ETIOLOGY	PREVALENCE
Group A streptococcus (GAS)	<18 y, 37%
	<5 y, 24%
Mycoplasma pneumoniae	5%–16%
Mononucleosis	Unknown

Source: Wald (2012).

TREATMENT

In developing a treatment plan, the challenge is twofold: (1) provide anticipatory guidance for a symptom-based plan and (2) educate the patient and caregiver on proper antibiotic use. The primary goal in treating the febrile patient is to improve comfort, not normalize temperature (Sullivan & Farrar, 2011). Increased fluid intake and reduced activity are the cornerstones of treatment for both children and adults with fever. The use of antipyretic medications may be given to a child who is uncomfortable, but detailed instructions on appropriate use, dosing measurement, and timing should be given to the parent. Sherman and Sood (2012) discuss the increasing toxicity of antipyretics, stating, "acetaminophen is the single leading medication implicated in pediatric emergency visits for drug overdose" (p. 402). Appropriate dosing for acetaminophen is 10 to 15 mg kg every 4 to 6 hours, with a maximum of 90 mg/kg over 24 hours, and not to exceed 2.6 g in 24 hours. Appropriate dosing for ibuprofen is 4 to 10 mg/kg every 6 to 8 hours, with a maximum of 40 mg/kg over 24 hours.

Anticipatory guidance on fever management should also include the following components (Ward, 2012):

- In otherwise healthy children, most fevers are self-limited and benign.
- Pushing fluids is recommended to maintain the patient's hydration status.
- Fever may merit treatment with an antipyretic agent if the child or adult is uncomfortable (e.g., decreased activity and decreased fluid intake).
- Acetaminophen is recommended as the starting medication because of its long track record of safety. There is insufficient evidence that alternating with ibuprofen is effective, and the practice may lead to dosing errors. In addition, the associated nephrotoxicity with ibuprofen negates its use in the dehydrated patient or those with renal insufficiency.
- Children who are receiving treatment for fever do not need to be awakened to receive the antipyretic agent.
- Children who are receiving antipyretic medications should not be given combination cough and cold preparations. Giving both medications may lead to inadvertent overdose.
- Antipyretic medication should be dosed according to the child's weight, not age.
- Information on the use of antipyretic medications should include written dosing instructions, the importance of using an approved measuring device, how to measure the appropriate volume, how often to administer, and how to monitor the response (Sullivan & Farrar, 2011).
- Aspirin should never be used to treat a child's fever because of the risk of Reye's syndrome.

Fever phobia and the perspective that a fever is harmful tend to contribute to the perceived need for antibiotics. In today's society, many believe that a fever equals an infection and an infection equals antibiotics. An explanation regarding the overuse of antibiotics and development of resistance may further assist the parent's understanding of why no prescription was written.

FOLLOW-UP

No visit is complete without providing explicit instructions for follow-up. Not only does this provide for patient and/or caregiver reassurance, it also helps mitigate the medico-legal risk. Research demonstrates variability for follow-up time but most studies suggest making contact with the family after 24 to 72 hours by either phone or in-person visit. Specific instruction should focus on warning signs and appropriate levels of care (primary care physician, pediatrician, urgent or emergency care). Stress to the parent that if there is ever a question with regard to the child's health, he or she should contact a health care professional.

Referrals

In cases where the child appears clinically ill (i.e., somnolent, dehydrated, and unresponsive) or in cases of febrile seizure, fever of more than 105°F, or unrelenting fever, the child should be referred to a high level of care. If you are in doubt as to the patient's health status, it is important to consult your collaborative physician or refer the child to another center.

ADULTS WITH FEVER

Assessment, diagnosis, and treatment of an adult fever do not vary much from those for children with a few exceptions. The threshold of concern for an adult fever is higher at 105.0°F. "Each increase of 1°F in temperature raises the basal metabolic rate by 7%, which results in increased demands on the heart" (Goroll & Mulley, 2006, p. 66). Use of antipyretic medications is recommended in adults with limited cardiac reserve.

CONCLUSION

Fever continues to be a challenging clinical situation for practitioners. Many myths and misconceptions perpetuate fear among patients, parents, and clinicians. Research shows that most acute fevers in children and adults are usually benign and self-limiting in nature. By reviewing the symptom in depth and using the helpful tools provided during visits, the clinician is better prepared to provide care for this common finding in the pediatric and adult populations.

10

Vital Signs: Recognizing and Managing Abnormalities

JILL JOHNSON, MARY C. HOMAN, AND
SANDRA F. RYAN

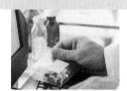

The assessment, measurement, and monitoring of a patient's vital signs are an important part of the physical examination and can provide an indication of the patient's overall well-being. Convenient care clinics (CCCs) play an important role in the early identification and accurate assessment of abnormal vital signs that can be risk factors for underlying illness and disease. The term "vital signs" is usually used to refer to the measurement of blood pressure (BP), heart rate, respiratory rate, and temperature. Pulse oximetry is known as the fifth vital sign. These five vital signs should be obtained in all acute visits—all are important in helping CCC providers determine appropriate diagnosis, treatment, and referrals.

In a convenient care setting, it is important from a quality of care and community health perspective to recognize and address abnormal vital signs. Abnormalities may require immediate action (e.g., hypertensive crisis) or nonurgent referrals (e.g., undiagnosed hypertension). However, abnormalities must also be considered in context; many factors can influence vital signs. Thorough patient history and examination are important when interpreting vital signs and overall clinical picture.

BLOOD PRESSURE

Blood pressure (BP) measurement is used in community chronic illness prevention; it is estimated that 29% to 31% of adults in the United States have hypertension, and many of them go undiagnosed (Egan, Zhao, & Axon, 2010).

Because a visit to a CCC may be the only encounter a patient has with a health care practitioner, screening in the clinic as part of routine visits can be life saving. In addition, many CCCs provide free drop-in BP checks as part of health promotion and disease prevention in the communities they serve.

Definitions and Etiologies

Key factors in accurate BP measurement

- Patient should be seated with both feet on the floor. Any movement can affect the accuracy of automated BP monitors; hence, ensure that patient remains still.
- The arm should be positioned at the level of the heart and well supported.
- Ideally, the patient should sit quietly for 5 minutes before taking the measurement. In the CCC setting, this should be true for taking a second measurement because the first reading was high.
  - Do take at least two readings on each visit if the first is elevated.
- Correct cuff size is essential for an accurate recording. The cuff should cover 100% of the circumference of the arm and two thirds of the length of the upper arm or lower leg with some overlap. The cuff bladder must cover 80% of the arm's circumference and be positioned over the artery. Incorrect cuff placement has been cited as a frequent source of error in both automated and manual BP measurement (Wedgbury & Valler-Jones, 2008).
- Inflate the bladder to 20 mmHg above systolic BP (SBP).
- Caffeine and smoking should be avoided for 1 hour before testing.

Normal BP is defined in adults as SBP less than 120 mmHg and diastolic BP (DBP) less than 80 mmHg. Hypotension is BP that is too low, and hypertension is BP that is too high. A distinction must be made between elevated BP as a finding and hypertension as a disease. One reading alone is not adequate to make a diagnosis of hypertension as a disease—this diagnosis requires at least two properly measured, seated BP readings on each of two or more office visits in patients who are not acutely ill. Some recommendations request three to six separate visits spaced over weeks to months to make a true diagnosis of new hypertension, primarily because of the concept of "white coat hypertension," anxiety about a provider visit that triggers increased BP—this phenomenon is found in up to 25% of patients with newly found elevated BP. Thus, relying on a single visit to diagnose hypertension will lead to over diagnosis and overtreatment.

When the SBP and DBP fall into different ranges, the highest category should be used to determine the stage of hypertension.

Elevated BP Emergencies

Elevated BP that causes symptoms such as headache, chest pain, blurred vision, or shortness of breath require emergent care. Hypertensive urgency is defined as SBP greater than 180 and/or DBP greater than 120 with no organ damage present. Hypertensive emergency is defined as a SBP greater than 180 and a DBP greater than 120 with organ damage occurring; hence, it is usually symptomatic. End organ damage can occur at lower BP levels and will usually be symptomatic. When symptoms are present or BP reaches urgent or emergent levels, patients should be referred to a higher level of care for further diagnostic testing and treatment. Although the BP does not need to be immediately lowered, patients do require urgent evaluation to determine the presence and extent of end organ damage.

Hypotension is when the BP is less than 90/60 mmHg. Because BP is related to size, age, hydration status, and medication use, it is more important to rely on symptoms than on absolute numbers. Orthostatic hypotension is defined as lowered BP or increased heart rate when a patient goes from a sitting to standing position. Numerically, an SBP decrease of at least 20 mmHg or a DBP decrease of at least 10 mmHg within 3 minutes of standing defines orthostatic hypotension (Bradley & Davis, 2003). Dizziness or lightheadedness when going from sitting to standing or lying to standing is also a sensitive sign. Orthostatic hypotension often represents volume depletion, and management and disposition should depend on the patient's ability to rehydrate.

Low BP Emergencies

Patients with symptomatic low BP may require emergent referral depending on the degree of symptoms, and judgment is needed. In cases where oral rehydration is difficult or sepsis is suspected, urgent or emergent referrals should be made.

MANAGING BLOOD PRESSURE ABNORMALITIES IN THE CCC

Elevated Blood Pressure

When elevated BP is detected, the provider's first step is to determine whether immediate action is needed because of possible end organ damage. If no immediate action is needed, the next step is to create a plan of action. The three most common presenting scenarios to a CCC are described below.

Elevated pressure during a visit for a typical CCC acute illness (e.g., sore throat or cough): Asymptomatic elevated BP can occur during any acute illness from (1) the underlying infectious process, (2) side effects of over-the-counter

Treatment of Hypertension

Lowering BP in patients with documented hypertension (persistently elevated on two to six repeat visits) will significantly lower the morbidity and mortality associated with heart failure, myocardial infarction, and stroke. Treatment should be based on lifestyle changes and medication therapy when warranted.

All patients with high BP should undergo lifestyle modifications including:

- Weight loss: Every kilogram of weight loss can result in a 2 mmHg drop in BP (Stevens et al., 1993)
- DASH diet (dietary approaches to stop hypertension): a low-fat, fiber-rich diet that is clinically proven to lower BP. Clear guidelines and patient information are published by the National Institutes of Health at http://www. nhlbi.nih.gov/health/public/heart/hbp/dash/new_dash.pdf
- Reduce dietary salt intake to no more than 2.4 g of sodium per day
- Limit alcohol consumption to no more than two drinks per day in men, one drink in women
- Exercise: at least 30 minutes of walking or more vigorous activity per day

Antihypertensives should be started in patients with proven stage 1 hypertension; two-drug therapy should be considered for patients with stage 2 hypertension. Although the target BP is 140/90, it may be lower in patients with risk factors for cardiovascular disease. Primary drugs used in monotherapy are thiazide diuretics, long-acting calcium channel blockers, and ACE inhibitors or angiotensin II receptor blockers. Combination therapy is used with two different agents when BP is persistently elevated despite monotherapy or in cases where BP is more than 20/10 mmHg above goal (Kaplan & Domino, 2012).

(OTC) medication for self-treatment, or (3) the abovementioned "white coat" syndrome. For these patients, take multiple readings during the same visit. Patients without a diagnosis of hypertension whose BP remains elevated during the first visit should be asked to return when they have recovered from their acute illness to have their BP rechecked. If patients show elevated BP during follow-up visits (two to six visits), they should be started on therapy (lifestyle changes, medication, or both) or referred to a primary care provider, depending on the clinic's policies. Patients with known but controlled hypertension should have their managing provider contacted to determine a joint treatment plan. During the acute illness, advise patients to avoid medications that can increase BP. Cases of patients with acute illness and apparent blood-pressure-related symptoms (e.g., severe headache in a patient with a urinary tract infection) should be treated as hypertensive emergencies.

Elevated BP identified during a screening or wellness examination: When hypertension is newly diagnosed, patients should receive a full workup including a baseline ECG and lab panel. In addition, causes of hypertension should be considered and ruled out. If this is not available in the CCC, or if continuity of care cannot be provided, patients should be referred nonurgently

Table 10.1 ■ **JNC 7—Classification of Blood Pressure for Adults**

CATEGORY	SBP (mmHg)		DBP (mmHg)
Hypotension	<90	and	<60
Normal	<120	and	<80
Pre-hypertensive	120–139	or	80–89
Hypertensive, stage 1	140–159	or	90–99

to a medical home. When treatment is warranted, the target measurement is BP of less than 140/90 mmHg.

Patient is aware of hypertension and has come for treatment: CCCs play an important role in helping to manage chronic disease because of their convenience and availability in the community. This is especially true for hypertension, which is controlled in fewer than 50% of patients. Patients who are already being treated for hypertension who present with elevated readings (as determined by an average of at least two measures per visit) should have therapeutic changes made in conjunction with their treating provider, provided that this is within the CCC's scope of practice. Patients who present with elevated BP but without a diagnosis of hypertension should return to the clinic for repeat testing (from two to six visits). If BP is consistently elevated, treatment should be initiated based on Joint National Committee (JNC 7) guidelines (see Table 10.1). Although there are many reasons hypertension is so poorly controlled, limited access to care plays a large role. Thus, in conjunction with local partners, CCCs play an important role in community high BP management. CCCs should have clear guidelines and policies around step therapy and medication algorithms.

Hypotension

Asymptomatic low BP needs to be understood in the context of the setting. If sepsis or underlying disease is suspected, low BP requires urgent referral. When hypotension is secondary to hypovolemia and the patient can tolerate oral rehydration, outpatient treatment with aggressive rehydration is appropriate. Providers should have a low threshold for referrals for symptomatic hypotension, particularly in the elderly (Bradley & Davis, 2003).

HYPERTENSION IN CHILDREN AND ADOLESCENTS

In children and adolescents, hypertension is defined as elevated BP that persists on repeated measurement at the 95th percentile or greater for age, height, and gender. Providers should be aware that hypertension can occur in children and that the incidence is on the rise.

Table 10.2 ■ Hypertension Criteria in Children and Adolescents

| AGE | GIRLS (SBP/DBP) | | BOYS (SBP/DBP) | |
	50TH PERCENTILE FOR HEIGHT	75TH PERCENTILE FOR HEIGHT	50TH PERCENTILE FOR HEIGHT	75TH PERCENTILE FOR HEIGHT
1	104/58	105/59	102/57	104/58
6	111/73	112/73	114/74	115/75
12	123/80	124/81	123/81	125/82
17	129/84	130/85	136/87	138/88

Adapted from National High Blood Pressure Education Program Working Group on Hypertension Control in Children and Adolescents (1996).

Table 10.2 provides the 95th percentile of BP according to age, gender, and the 50th and 75th height percentiles in children and adolescents. In general, persistently elevated BP in pediatric patients should be referred to a pediatrician.

HEART RATE

Many factors can affect a patient's heart rate, such as illness, pain, emotional stress, current fitness level, medications, age, body size, and body position. Heart rate is a vital component of the patient's vital signs and should be measured on every acute visit. Rate should be measured for 1 minute and reported as beats per minute. Normal heart rates are

- Children (1–10 years): 70 to 130 bpm
- Children older than 10 years through adult: 60 to 100 bpm
- Well-trained and conditioned athletes: 40 to 60 bpm

Tachycardia is defined as fast heart rate, whereas bradycardia is an abnormally low rate. The majority of tachycardia can be explained in context of the presenting illness including fever, dehydration, or over-the-counter (OTC) use. It can also be a harbinger of more serious diagnoses such as hyperthyroidism, sepsis, heart failure, pulmonary embolism, or hypoxia. Bradycardia can be due to acute illness, medication or drug use, or cardiac disease. Symptomatic tachycardia (lightheadedness, chest pain, and palpitations) or bradycardia (lightheadedness and syncope) should be referred for treatment or further evaluation. In addition, significantly elevated heart rates should have a low threshold for referral for further diagnostic testing.

TEMPERATURE

Fluctuations in body temperature occur naturally in everyone as a result of circadian rhythms, age, exertion, and hormonal balance. Low and high body temperatures in adults and children can have significant implications.

- Normal range of body temperature is 96.8°F to 99.5°F (36°C to 37.5°C) depending on the site measured.
- In children, temperature above the following levels is considered a fever:
  Rectally: 100.4°F (38°C)
  Orally: 99.5°F (37.5°C)
  Axillary: 99°F (37.2°C)
- In an adult, temperature above 99 to 99.5°F (37.2–37.5°C), depending on the time of day, can indicate fever.

Accurate Measurement

All noninvasive temperature measurement methods vary in accuracy; rectal readings are considered the most accurate reflection of a body's core temperature (Bridges & Thomas, 2009). In the convenient care setting, oral temperatures are the next best option. Oral and temporal artery temperature measurements were found to be more precise than axillary and tympanic measurements (ENA, 2011).

Temperature Abnormalities

Hypothermia is temperature below 95°F/35°C and can occur when the body's mechanisms to create heat are ineffective. Examples of potential causes include cold exposure, metabolic imbalances, substance intoxication or use, sepsis, or deterioration of physiological functions. Patients with symptomatic hypothermia should be sent to the emergency department for further evaluation.

Hyperthermia is temperature above 99.5°F/37.5°C. Causes of hyperthermia include infections, medications, central nervous system insults, multisystem responses, and environmental factors. Patients presenting with fever will generally respond to antipyretics (acetaminophen and ibuprofen), treatment of the underlying disease, and increased fluid intake. Pediatric patients with fever who are not taking fluids, have decreased urine output, or appear lethargic need to be sent to the emergency department. Acutely ill patients with fever higher than 103°F/39.4°C will often require further diagnostic testing.

Table 10.3 ■ Normal Respiration Rates by Age

AGE GROUP	NORMAL
Infants	20–40 breaths per minute
Children	20–30 breaths per minute
Adults	12–20 breaths per minute

RESPIRATION

Normal respiratory rate (i.e., eupnea) varies with age and is influenced by activities, illness, emotions, and medications. Respiratory rate should be assessed for all acute illness visits presenting at a CCC. The average respiratory to pulse rate is 1:4, that is, 1 respiration to 4 pulse beats. Respirations should be counted for at least 30 seconds and then doubled. If respirations are irregular, count for the full 1 minute to get an accurate measure. Table 10.3 shows normal respiration rates.

Red Flags and Differential Diagnoses

A raised or decreased respiratory rate can be a strong and specific predictor of a serious adverse event or underlying condition. Although there is no one finding that mandates emergent or urgent referral, the symptoms listed below may warrant such referral. When respiratory distress accompanies respiratory rate abnormalities, patients should be referred for more urgent care elsewhere.

- Rate greater than 40 respirations per minute
- Skin color, pallor, mottling, cyanosis, and any petechial rash around the eyelids, face, and neck may indicate a possible oxygenation problem
- Infants and children younger than age 7 are predominantly abdominal breathers; anything affecting the abdomen may interfere with their breathing and oxygenation
- Signs of respiratory distress (e.g., nasal flaring, grunting, wheezing, stridor, dyspnea, and use of accessory muscles)

Pulse Oximetry

Pulse oximetry entails using a spectrophotometric device to establish the oxygen saturation levels in a patient's hemoglobin. To estimate saturation over a wide range of pulse volumes, the pulse oximeter automatically increases its amplification as the pulse signal decreases.

- Normal pulse oximetry (SpO$_2$) is 95% or greater
- SpO$_2$ of 92% or less (at sea level) suggests hypoxemia
- The accuracy of the pulse oximeter is within ±2% to ±3% when a patient's oxygen saturation is 90% or greater

In a patient with acute respiratory illness (e.g., influenza) or breathing difficulty (e.g., asthma attack), an SpO$_2$ of 92% or less indicates the possible need for oxygen or treatment.

In a patient with stable chronic disease (e.g., chronic obstructive pullmonary disease [COPD]), an SpO$_2$ of 92% or less should prompt referral for further evaluation for long-term oxygen therapy, to the emergency room if SpO$_2$ is unstable or to the primary care provider if stable.

Key Factors in Accurate Pulse Oximetry

- Research supports that a pulse oximeter probe should be attached only to the intended site and should be the correct size (adult and pediatric). Placing a pulse oximeter finger sensor on an ear or an adult sensor on a pediatric patient does not provide a reliable measurement (Haynes, 2007).
- Nail polish (especially dark shades) and artificial nails can affect accuracy of the measurement.
- Accurate oxygen measurement requires a good blood flow through the tissues. Cold hands and fingers or poor perfusion result in poor or inaccurate readings.
- Movement may interfere with accuracy.
- If there is doubt about the accuracy of a reading, the probe should be tested on the practitioner's finger or ear lobe.

CONCLUSION

By obtaining accurate vital signs, CCCs can play an instrumental role in identifying problems or risks. Vital signs are one component of the overall visit, and each vital sign should be looked at independently as well as collectively with the overall clinical picture when making diagnoses and treating, referring, and counseling patients. CCCs and the health care providers who staff them are in a unique position to utilize vital signs to promote health and prevent diseases in children and adults.

11

Sports Physicals: The Preparticipation Physical Evaluation

SUSAN M. COOLEY, ELIZABETH PERIUS, AND KEVIN RONNEBERG

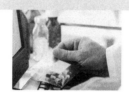

Sports physicals, known as preparticipation physical evaluations (PPEs), are an important service provided by nurse practitioners (NPs) and physician assistants (PAs) in retail-based convenient care settings. Required PPEs are one of the most common reasons teens seek primary care (Greene, 2000), and these examinations offer an important opportunity to evaluate their general health and provide preventive counseling.

The overarching goal in performing a PPE is to promote safe participation in sports and physical activity (Bernhardt & Roberts, 2010). The PPE is an effective tool in identifying medical and orthopedic conditions that could affect the athlete's ability to safely participate in sports. Although no evidence exists that demonstrates that PPEs detect life-threatening conditions, they do screen for abnormalities that predispose the athlete to injury, illness, or sudden death (Bernhardt & Roberts, 2010).

Sports participation for athletes with special needs provides the same benefits as for athletes without special needs: increased endurance, muscle strength, and flexibility, and improved cardiovascular function, balance, and motor skills. In addition, sports participation is associated with increased self-esteem and reduced anxiety and depression (Bernhardt & Roberts, 2010). Although some athletes with special needs may require consultation with a primary care provider or specialist, it is important to facilitate a PPE for these patients.

ADMINISTRATION

The ideal timing of a PPE is 6 to 8 weeks before beginning the sport, providing ample time for further evaluation or rehabilitation of any problems discovered during the examination and thus preventing other injuries. The length of time between evaluations varies across athletic departments.

Typically athletes present to the clinic with the required forms for their school. This form is an invaluable tool with targeted risk assessment questions. The medical history portion should be completed by the athlete and parent before the visit and reviewed with the health care provider during the evaluation. If a patient arrives with no form, a standard PPE form may be available to download from the athlete's athletic department or state high school athletic association website. The National Federation of State High School Associations (www.nfhs.org) provides links to state association member sites.

The Health Insurance Portability and Accountability Act of 1996 privacy rules allow release of medical information in certain circumstances. The recommendation to clear the participant or not may be provided to coaches and school administration officials without an individual's authorization. More detailed information about the medical reason for nonclearance requires a signed authorization for release of patient information (Bernhardt & Roberts, 2010).

HISTORY

The most important element of the PPE is the collection and review of thorough personal and family medical histories (Bernhardt & Roberts, 2010). This is best achieved in the presence of a parent or guardian with lifelong knowledge of the athlete (Bernhardt & Roberts, 2010). Sudden cardiac death (SCD), occurring in approximately 1 of 200,000 young athletes, is the most serious condition for which athletes are screened (Giese, O'Connor, Brennan, Depenbrock, & Oriscello, 2007). The history may be the only way to reveal potential problems because many of the conditions that may precipitate SCD may have normal physical findings (Giese et al., 2007). The primary abnormalities contributing to SCD are hypertrophic cardiomyopathy and coronary artery anomalies (Giese et al., 2007). The American Heart Association (AHA) recommends referral for the following five historical items: exertional chest pain or discomfort, unexplained syncope or near syncope, excessive exertional or unexplained dyspnea or fatigue, heart murmur, and elevated blood pressure (Maron et al., 2007). Red flags in the family history requiring further evaluation to determine eligibility for sports participation include sudden death before age 50, early coronary artery disease or anomalies, hypertrophic cardiomyopathy, lethal arrhythmias, or Marfan syndrome (Giese et al., 2007; Greene, 2000; Maron et al., 2007).

Review major and recent injuries and illnesses, such as dizziness or collapse with exertion and heat-related events, that usually indicate need for referral. Athletes with a history of multiple concussions need further evaluation to determine risk associated with continued contact sports. "Burners/stingers" result from trauma to the head or neck, causing unilateral pain, numbness, and/or tingling in the shoulder or arm (Bernhardt & Roberts, 2010). A history of bilateral pain, numbness, and/or tingling or repeated stingers could indicate spinal cord pathology and warrants further evaluation (Bernhardt & Roberts, 2010).

Information about current medications, allergies, anaphylaxis, immunizations, hospitalizations, surgeries, fractures, and menstrual history for female patients ensures a complete history. Functional history regarding organs such as eyes, testicles, and kidneys should be obtained; dysfunction in one of a paired organ is a risk factor for total functional loss and warrants referral. Use of eyeglasses, contact lenses, or dental braces should be noted, as the athlete may need protective wear to avoid injury.

PHYSICAL EXAMINATION

A PPE should be performed when the patient is not ill, thus avoiding any unnecessary restrictions on activity. Adolescents should be seen apart from their parents or guardians for at least part of the examination to allow the clinician to inquire about risk-taking behaviors. It is important to set the stage for this early in the evaluation. Privacy is of utmost importance for the examination and counseling of both male and female patients.

Obtain vital signs including blood pressure, pulse, height, weight, and body mass index (BMI), and visual acuity. A standard head-to-toe assessment with a brief musculoskeletal assessment is required. Most conditions that warrant referral are identified through the cardiac and the musculoskeletal examinations (Small, 2009).

The AHA guidelines suggest referral for one or more of the following findings on physical examination: heart murmur, diminished femoral pulses, features associated with Marfan syndrome, or hypertension (Maron et al., 2007). Cardiac auscultation should be obtained both sitting and supine to increase the likelihood of detecting a heart murmur (Giese et al., 2007). Some characteristics of pathological murmurs include loudness (grade III or higher), long duration (mid or late peak or a holosystolic murmur), diastolic murmur, changes in intensity with position changes, or a murmur noted in the presence of other heart sounds (Giese et al., 2007). Systolic ejection murmurs are associated with aortic stenosis. Other common causes of sudden death in athletes may or may not be associated with a heart murmur (Giese et al., 2007). Some defining characteristics in Marfan syndrome are pectus excavatum, joint hyperextensibility, arm span greater than height, or a murmur (associated with aortic or mitral valve insufficiency; Giese et al., 2007). Hypertension, using pediatric age-based parameters, warrants referral to a primary care provider.

The musculoskeletal examination is a brief, focused assessment of joint range of motion, muscular strength, deformities, and coordination (see Table 11.1). Abnormalities should be referred for further evaluation. The Two-Minute Musculoskeletal Examination described in Table 11.1 can be conducted efficiently with a negative patient history.

Table 11.1 ■ **Two-Minute Musculoskeletal Examination**

1. Patient facing examiner: note general body habitus. Observe for symmetry of trunk and upper extremities
2. Assess cervical spine range of motion: instruct patient to look at ceiling, floor, over both shoulders, and touch ears to shoulders
3. Assess shoulder function with shoulder shrug with examiner resistance. Assess trapezoid and deltoid strength
4. Shoulder (glenohumeral joint) ROM (range of motion) assessed with internal and external rotation
5. Elbow ROM assessed with extension and flexion
6. Evaluate hands for rotational deformities by asking the patient to open and close the fists and spread apart fingers
7. Assess back and upper extremities with patient facing away from examiner
8. Observe spine flexibility: have patient stand, knees straight, back extended, and chin tilted toward the ceiling
9. Scoliosis examination: bend forward, with knees straight, touch toes, observe for spine curvature/rib-hump
10. Four-step "duck walk" toward examiner will assess hip, knee, and ankle function as well as strength and balance
11. Observe patient doing toe/heel raises for calf strength and balance

Adapted from Uphold and Graham (2003a).

The head, ears, eyes, nose, and throat examination, in addition to the standard physical examination, includes noting pupil size equality. Documentation of anisocoria, present in 20% of the population, becomes important in the event of a future head injury (MedlinePlus, 2011). Abnormal lung sounds (e.g., wheezing) should be treated and/or referred for further evaluation. Abnormal abdominal findings including tenderness, organomegaly, hernia, or distention require referral. Tanner stage should be assessed and noted. All male PPEs require an external genitourinary examination to assess for inguinal hernia, undescended testicle, hydrocele, varicocele, or maturation abnormalities. The skin examination is important to reduce the spread of infectious dermatoses such as impetigo, tinea, and herpes during contact sports such as wrestling. The PPE also provides an opportunity to discuss acne treatment.

HEALTH EDUCATION OPPORTUNITY

The PPE is an excellent opportunity to provide preventive counseling and health and safety guidance for both the teen and the parent/guardian. Time restraints may limit the amount of counseling during the PPE; choose topics pertinent to the individual based on the history obtained. Topics might include the following:

1. Safety (including seatbelt use and safe driving, helmets and other protective equipment, and personal safety through awareness of the surrounding environment)
2. Proper rest and hydration promote a healthy athletic performance

3. Children with elevated BMI should be counseled along with their parent(s) on strategies for healthy nutrition and regular exercise
4. Sun protection, especially if the teen will be engaging in an outdoor sport
5. Anabolic steroid avoidance (undesirable side effects of acne and atrophy of breasts/testicles may be a deterrent to the approximately 500,000 high school students using them; U.S. DOJ, 2004)
6. Tobacco, alcohol, and drug use are pervasive in American society and should be addressed in any teen health visit
7. Breast and testicular self-examination (6% of testicular cancers are found in males under age 20; National Cancer Institute, 2012)
8. Abstinence or condom use should be encouraged to prevent pregnancy and transmission of HIV and other sexually transmitted infections

CLEARANCE FOR PARTICIPATION

National data show that fewer than 2% of patients are disqualified from sports participation (Rice, 2010). Sports vary by level of contact and cardiac static/dynamic demand. When an abnormality is detected, the type of sport and severity of the abnormality must be taken into consideration when making the determination regarding the athlete's participation in that sport. Table 11.2 shows common sports by level of contact required during play. Table 11.3 shows sports classification according to the cardiovascular demand achieved during competition.

Table 11.2 ■ Classification of Common Sports According to Contact

CONTACT/COLLISION	LIMITED CONTACT	NONCONTACT
Basketball	Baseball	Badminton
Boxing	White-water rafting	Bodybuilding
Cheerleading	Fencing	Bowling
Field hockey	High jump, pole-vault	Dance
Football, tackle	Football–flag or touch	Golf
Gymnastics	Softball	Sailing
Lacrosse	Volleyball	Swimming
Soccer	Weight lifting	Tennis
Wrestling	Track	

Adapted from Bernhardt and Roberts (2010).

Table 11.3 ■ Classification of Sports According to Cardiovascular Demands

LOW DYNAMIC/ LOW STATIC	LOW DYNAMIC/ HIGH STATIC	HIGH DYNAMIC/ LOW STATIC	HIGH DYNAMIC/ HIGH STATIC
Bowling	Archery	Basketball	Boxing
Riflery	Gymnastics	Lacrosse	Water polo
Golf	Weight lifting	Soccer	Wrestling
	Water skiing	Volleyball	Football
	Rodeo	Racquetball	Downhill skiing

Adapted from Bernhardt and Rogers (2010).

Table 11.4 ■ Medical Condition, Participations, and Referral for Further Evaluation

MAY NOT PLAY	MAY PLAY	NEED FURTHER EVALUATION	
Carditis	Asthma—controlled	Heart murmur	Seizures—poorly controlled
Fever	Diabetes—controlled	Congenital heart disease	Cerebral palsy
Acute splenomegaly	Seizure disorder-controlled	Hypertension	Musculoskeletal disorder
Moderate to severe diarrhea	Innocent murmur	Single functional eye/kidney	Pulmonary disease
	HIV	History of heat illness	Eating disorders—anorexia/bulimia
	Sickle cell	History of head or spinal injury	Atlantoaxial instability
	Single ovary or testicle	Contagious skin lesions	Kidney disease—hydronephrosis
	Obesity	Bleeding disorders	Mild diarrhea
		Acute musculoskeletal injury	

Adapted from Bernhardt and Roberts (2010).

Clearance levels generally fall into one of four categories: (1) unrestricted participation in any sport, including contact sports with high dynamic/static demands, (2) clearance with restrictions that apply to the athlete needing special treatment during play (e.g., a patient with well-controlled mild to moderate exercise-induced asthma), (3) deferred clearance pending further workup of a condition found on either the history or physical examination, such as heart murmur or concussion, and (4) not cleared because a patient's condition precludes participation in a particular sport. Patients seen in a convenient care clinic (CCC) setting with a clearance level other than unrestricted require a referral. See Table 11.4 for specific conditions that merit referral.

REFERRALS

CCC operators must establish clear protocols for referral to appropriate primary care providers or specialists for coordination of further evaluation, treatment, or remediation for every patient who is not cleared for participation. The clinician should assist in making arrangements for follow-up for patients who do not have a primary physician, including low-income and uninsured patients. When making a referral for further workup, it is important that a summary of findings as well as a clear explanation of the reason for referral be provided to the patient and parent.

SUMMARY

NPs and PAs working in convenient care settings provide an excellent resource for patients in need of annual PPEs. Retail-based convenient care has gained popularity with health care consumers as a resource for these services because of its convenience, accessibility, lower prices, and documented high-quality services (Weinick, Pollack, Fisher, Gillen, & Mehrotra, 2010). Standardization of the PPE process allows for appropriate assessment and referral of the patient. Collaboration between convenient care providers and school personnel can give parents options for the PPE. Referral for evaluation and coordination of care ensures the best possible outcome when abnormal findings are encountered on the PPE. Collaboration with the primary care provider provides continuity and quality of care for the athlete.

12

Specific Populations in the Convenient Care Clinic Setting

TANIA CELIA AND SANDRA F. RYAN

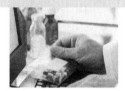

In every health care setting, there are special populations of patients who have unique needs. The convenient care clinic (CCC) setting is no exception, with clinic providers seeing patients from 18 months to elderly for acute conditions, screenings, and routine preventive care. In this chapter, we will review two very important groups of people who are responsible for a large number of visits in health care: pediatrics and geriatrics. This chapter reviews the physiological and psychological changes that occur within these groups to help providers with their interactions with these populations and to manage their care.

PEDIATRICS

Providing health care to children requires providers to have an in-depth understanding of the pediatric developmental stages. Providers will use this knowledge not only when interacting with the pediatric patient but also when giving anticipatory guidance to the child's parent. In the convenient care setting, providers have the ability to use every pediatric encounter to assess developmental issues such as proper growth, speech development, and immunization status.

DEVELOPMENTAL STAGES/PHYSIOLOGIC CHANGES OVERVIEW

Infant to 12 Months

Infants are children from birth to 12 months. They require careful supervision and monitoring for any health issues, and parents need anticipatory guidance, reassurance, and teaching to know what to expect as their child grows. Infants undergo rapid growth and development in their first year of life and require frequent visits to their pediatric health care providers. This age group is not seen in the CCC setting at present and will not be further addressed in this chapter.

Toddler (12 to 36 Months)

Toddlers are children who are about 1 to 3 years old. This is a challenging time for parents—children are developing their independence, identity, and motor skills but have little regard for any sense of danger (Mills & Woodring, 2012). Toddlers about 12 months of age are generally still working on walking, self-feeding, pointing to objects, and developing a limited vocabulary (Uphold & Graham, 2003). At 15 to 18 months, their abilities continue to expand. By the time children are about 18 months old, they start to run and they have a larger vocabulary (Uphold & Graham, 2003b).

Physically, growth is still rapid but slower than during infancy. The head changes, and its size becomes more proportional to the rest of the body, while the arms and legs lengthen. Toddlers typically have a potbelly appearance, but this dissipates as chest circumference increases. Vital signs change, with pulse and respiratory rate decreasing during this time while blood pressure increases to become more in line with adult values. Vision is still not fully developed and will not be 20/20 until the preschool years. Toddlers are infamous for their picky food choices. This is actually related to changes in the necessary caloric intake, which decreases with the slowed growth during this time. By age 3, most children have all of their primary teeth as well. Another task for toddlers to accomplish is toilet training, which is often accompanied by exploration of the body (Mills & Woodring, 2012).

Children during the toddler years typically display some separation anxiety and fear of strangers, but this dissipates as they age. Tantrums in this age group are very common and considered a rite of passage; children have increasing independence and test their limitations. It is recommended that health care providers working with children of this age group address issues directly using age-appropriate vocabulary. Because these children normally have a decreased attention span, short and simple explanations are best. Meeting toddlers at their eye level and using play to help them understand what the office visit may entail makes it less intimidating for them. Using terms that can be misinterpreted literally is generally not recommended because this can lead to confusion for the child (Mills & Woodring, 2012).

CCCs begin to see toddlers between 18 and 24 months of age.

Preschool (3 to 6 Years)

Children in their preschool years undergo multiple physical changes. Visual acuity should mature to 20/20 with concurrent improvement in hand–eye coordination. Children gain an average of 3 inches in height and 5 pounds yearly. Because the musculoskeletal system needs additional fuel for the extensive growth of muscle and bones, nutrition is a concern as well. Children have all of their primary teeth and may begin to lose some of them by the time they are of school age (Reynolds, 2012).

Children learn activities of daily living at this time, such as how to dress and feed themselves. Feeding habits tend to change as growth waxes and wanes. Usually preschoolers have developed bowel and bladder control but may continue to have nighttime issues. Preschool children must also learn to socialize more as they begin school. This age group begins to learn right from wrong and the concept of there being consequences for their inappropriate actions, such as punishments. Reinforcement of what is expected in terms of appropriate behavior is needed often (Reynolds, 2012).

Preschool children often develop fear of both real and make-believe things; in some cases, it may be simply fear of the dark or a fear of monsters. It is recommended to deal with children's fears realistically but also not to force them to confront their fears (Reynolds, 2012). It is also recommended to allow children to make choices when appropriate while at the same time avoiding power struggles (Uphold & Graham, 2003).

School (6 to 12 Years)

Children of this age group are eager to test their boundaries but still tend not to make good decisions. For this reason, safety must be emphasized at this age. Friends become more of an interest and children gradually migrate toward them (Uphold & Graham, 2003). School-age children generally have consistent, steady growth and add 7 pounds per year on average, while their height increases about 2.5 inches per year (Feigleman as cited in O'Connor-Von, 2012). As school-age children grow, muscle strength and size increase, which correlates with an improvement in gross motor skills (O'Connor-Von, 2012). Biometric measures also change in this age group; the heart grows in size and the heart rate drops. Most children of this group have an average apical pulse of about 90 beats per minute, and the respiratory rate also drops at this time, approaching 20 breaths per minute (O'Connor-Von, 2012). Children of this age group have often been exposed to the majority of childhood illnesses and tend to get sick less. Interestingly, the immune system matures and antibodies such as IgG and IgA reach adult levels around age 7 (O'Connor-Von, 2012). Advancing verbal skills make communication easier in this age group, and comprehension and verbal expression also gradually build. At the high end of this age range, there is an increased understanding of conversation other than the literal translation of words (O'Connor-Von, 2012). Health care providers interacting with this age group will often find them inquisitive and interactive.

Adolescence (12 to 18 Years)

Adolescence is a unique time in life where a young person is halfway between childhood and adulthood. Often the body of an adolescent will mature before emotional development is complete. Adolescence is characterized by a growth spurt during which boys can expect to grow up to 6 inches and add up to 15 pounds and girls can grow up to 5 inches and add up to 10 pounds on average. The growth spurt often begins with weight and can extend over a period of several years. Growth during this time is accompanied by the onset of puberty, and rapid growth and the development of secondary sex characteristics can be a source of embarrassment for the adolescent (Mandelco & McCoy, 2012).

Most adolescents have a teenage mind in an adult body. Because peer influence is so strong in this group, often adolescents will consider friends' opinions carefully. Appearance is of the utmost importance. Teen girls are at a risk of developing eating disorders if they perceive themselves to be overweight, or their peers do. Adolescents are also prone to risk-taking behaviors, and this can often involve motor vehicle accidents as they become new drivers. Asserting independence is a task of this age group as teens begin to consider long-term goals. It is increasingly important to counsel adolescents on drug and alcohol use and the risks of sexually transmitted infections. Because the average age of the onset of puberty is now about age 12, it is important to start this conversation early, before children get too far into this developmental stage (Uphold & Graham, 2003).

PRESCRIBING IN THE PEDIATRIC POPULATION

Children differ significantly from adults in terms of physiology and, thus, prescribing for children will differ from doing so for adults. Among other considerations, providers must factor in that many medications have not been tested in this population before use (Novak & Allen, 2007). In the recent past, labeling requirements were only necessary in most cases for adult medication usage, and there was very little labeling or testing for pediatric patients (Wilson as cited in Novak & Allen, 2007). This resulted in Congress passing two pieces of legislation in the past several years: the Best Pharmaceuticals for Children Act in 2002 and the Pediatric Research Equity Act in 2003. These acts encourage more research before using medications in the pediatric population and also resulted in changing the labeling for many medications (including many over-the-counter medications) (Clarke, 2011). It is essential that providers consider the differences in pediatric patients' absorption, elimination, metabolism, and distribution when prescribing (Novak & Allen, 2007). In addition, the provider should consider comorbidities, interactions, the child's development, and other medications being used concurrently (Adcock as cited in Novak & Allen, 2007). Weight-based dosing is a standard of pediatric care, and with the increasing number of obese children who are being seen in primary care, this must also be considered. Even with obese children, providers must be sure to stay within acceptable established ranges of safety for any medication (Adcock as cited in Novak & Allen, 2007).

Long-Term Considerations

The past few decades have seen the development of chronic diseases in pediatric patients—previously seen only in adults—which has dramatically changed the management of these children in primary care.

Every encounter that a provider has with a pediatric patient should address growth and development issues. As noted, obesity among children is increasing at an alarming rate (Miller & Silverstein, 2006), resulting in the development of multiple chronic health issues in pediatric patients, which were previously seen only in adults. Sleep apnea, cardiovascular disease, and impaired glucose tolerance are just a few of the issues that are now being found in pediatric patients as a result of obesity (Must as cited in Miller & Silverstein, 2006). If these issues are not corrected, they can persist into the adult years. Miller and Silverstein (2006) state that these chronic health issues also increase the burden on the country's medical resources as the number of people with chronic health problems increases. Clearly this is an issue that cannot be ignored, and CCC providers can play an important role in addressing obesity in children and educating their parents, who may not realize its long-reaching effects.

GERIATRICS

According to the United States Department of Health and Human Services, the elderly (those older than 65) are the fastest-growing part of our population; the current level is expected to blossom to 72 million elderly by the year 2030 (2011, as cited in Shah & Hajjar, 2012). This means that we will continue to see more elderly patients in all health care settings, and there is a good chance that they will develop more chronic medical conditions. Special consideration and understanding of the geriatric patient's needs will help ensure quality health care delivery.

Physiological Changes

It is important to remember that our bodies change as we age and that these changes can affect how our bodies respond to illness. Rughwani (2011) details multiple changes that occur as we age.

In the cardiovascular area, both the body's reduced response to adrenaline during physical stress and the decrease in variability of the heart rate can be concerning (Rughwani, 2011). Cefalu (2011) states that there is an up to 90% reduction in the cells of the sinus node that control the body's heart rate as we age, resulting in lower heart rates at rest and during periods of stress. The increased peripheral vascular resistance that is seen with aging has long been associated with hypertension in the elderly (Rughwani, 2011). Thus, we need to carefully use our assessment skills with these patients; the potential exists for the elderly to be very ill yet have vital signs that do not reflect the extent of their illness. The increased vascular resistance should also be considered carefully when we are prescribing medications.

The respiratory system undergoes multiple important age-related changes. Cefalu (2011) states that our lung function generally starts to decrease after age 25 and continues to worsen over time. There are fewer alveoli in the lung tissue, and there is less flexibility of the lungs and diminished ciliary action (Rughwani, 2011). In addition, there are smaller numbers of receptors in the airways as we age, which affects how we respond to medications (Cefalu, 2011). If we combine this with weaker respiratory muscles, an increase in the number of bronchial mucus glands, and decreased mobility in the chest wall (Rughwani, 2011), we have good reason to be concerned. This combination of factors results in a weaker cough, an increased risk for infections, and reduced ability to clear secretions. This puts the older adult at higher risk for pneumonia, which can be devastating in this age group.

Because of age-related changes in the liver, there is less blood flow, which means there is decreased ability for the body to detoxify itself (Rughwani, 2011). This reduced detoxification is true of normal body waste as well as drugs and supplements. In addition, the oxidation and reduction phases lead to impaired metabolism, which specifically affects the breakdown of benzodiazepines (Cefalu, 2011). The kidneys have a similar issue; the lower blood perfusion to the kidneys results in a decreased glomerular filtration rate and creatinine clearance, which in turn interferes with the body's ability to clear medication and other toxins that are broken down by the kidneys (Rughwani, 2011). As health care providers, we need to be extremely cautious with medication regimens for our elderly patients and should try to use the least amount of medication that is still effective.

The immune system also changes significantly as we age. There are fewer naïve T cells, and function of B cells and T cells is reduced (Rughwani, 2011); this means that the immune system is slower to respond to infections. Illness can be very advanced in elderly patients before they show an immune response, and it takes much longer for these patients to develop an immune response to infectious processes.

The increase in the aging population also means that there has been an increase in complex, chronic illnesses that our patients are living with daily. The Centers for Disease Control and Prevention (2003, as cited in Shah & Hajjar, 2012) estimates that over three-quarters of the elderly have a minimum of one chronic health problem that requires several medications to manage adequately, and about half have two or more. This results in an increase in medication-related issues and potential for patients to be taking more medications than necessary.

CONCLUSION

As the nation ages, we will see more elderly patients looking for convenient, quality health care. CCCs and the providers who staff them are in a great position to help ensure that the needs of the geriatric population are met and that these patients are receiving appropriate screening, counseling, and medication reconciliation.

13

Vaccinations in the Convenient Care Clinic

BARBARA SPYCHALLA AND SANDRA F. RYAN

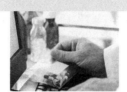

Immunizations are the number-one way to prevent disease and promote health. Convenient care clinics (CCCs) provide a convenient access point and an excellent opportunity for individuals to receive needed immunizations. Although there is some debate about the role of CCCs in routine pediatric immunization, the clinics offer numerous benefits related to vaccinations and immunizations.

- In most states, students must have up-to-date immunizations before they can enroll in school. CCCs can provide these "catch-up" vaccines efficiently and conveniently.
- Employers, particularly employers of health care workers, often require certain vaccinations before employment, and CCCs can provide these.
- Flu shots: One of the most common vaccines administered in CCCs is the influenza vaccine to prevent flu. In fact, anecdotal information from one CCC reports that up to 90% of shoppers who received a flu vaccine were not planning to get one that day but received it after seeing in-store signs. Flu shots are a true "impulse buy."

CCCs commonly offer vaccines against herpes zoster, pneumococcal disease, hepatitis A and B, tetanus, diphtheria, pertussis, meningitis, human papilloma virus, measles/mumps/rubella, and varicella.

HOW ARE WE DOING AS A NATION?

Improving vaccination rates has been a long-term goal of quality improvement and regulatory bodies. Vigilance toward immunization of children and adults is addressed by the Office of Disease Prevention and Health Promotion in *Healthy People 2010*. These target objectives are proposed to be retained in

Healthy People 2020 because the objectives from 2010 have not been met. For example, the *Healthy People 2010* target for pneumococcal vaccine in adults aged 65 years and older is 90%. As of 2008, studies showed that only 60% of that population was immunized (Lu & Nuorti, 2010). Vaccine-preventable disease rates in the United States are at low levels for measles, rubella, diphtheria, polio, and tetanus (World Health Organization, 2012); however, because of waning immunity and lower immunization rates, some preventable diseases are making a comeback, such as pertussis. As demonstrated during the flu season of 2009 to 2010 with the outbreak of H1N1 influenza, we cannot afford complacency in our attitudes toward vaccines and vaccination. Because many patients do not have a primary care provider, each visit to a CCC should be an opportunity to promote prevention and immunizations.

PROMOTING HEALTH ONE VISIT AT A TIME

All health care providers must be committed to addressing immunization status at every visit and advocating the necessary vaccines for preventing disease and promoting patient health. Providers must be knowledgeable about and willing to address and dispel barriers and public beliefs that prevent patients from receiving needed immunizations. Inconvenient locations and hours, cost, and misconceptions about safety are just a few known barriers to immunizing. There are various barriers to immunizations, but none are insurmountable. Some of these barriers include:

Missed opportunities: Health care providers should address vaccination needs for both adults and children at each visit or encounter. The Centers for Disease Control and Prevention (CDC) relates that studies have shown that eliminating missed opportunities could increase vaccination coverage by up to 20%.

Provider misconceptions: Education of providers regarding vaccinations—contraindications, schedules, and simultaneous vaccine administration—is imperative for achieving improved immunity to vaccine-preventable diseases in child and adult populations. Providers must be advocates for vaccine administration to promote health and prevent disease. Patients who receive information from a trusted health care professional such as a nurse practitioner are more likely to act on the advice given.

Patient misconceptions: The nature of the CCC is such that many patients represent the generation of the "young and invincible"; many others have just never been affected by the disease that a particular vaccine prevents (e.g., influenza) and do not believe they need it. Whatever the reason, many CCC patients believe that they are invulnerable to the diseases that vaccinations prevent. Thus, it is extremely important for providers to share with their patients the value of prevention and the benefits of vaccination, one particular benefit being "herd immunity," the concept of protecting of the individual through the benefits of the "herd." That is, those who have been vaccinated do not tend to become infected and hence cannot pass on the illness to others, and this protects those who, for example, cannot receive vaccinations because of contraindications or those in whom the disease is most impactful (such as the very young and the very old). It is the clinician's responsibility to let patients know that vaccinations are not only good for the patient but also good for the community.

Parents believe that their children are fully vaccinated when they are not: It is important to provide vaccination records/vaccine history and return dates at every vaccination encounter, and to inquire about vaccination status at every visit, regardless of the chief complaint. Parents should be encouraged to carry their child's vaccine record with them to every health care visit. Records of immunizations should include the type of vaccine given (manufacturer and lot number), date, dose, site, route of administration, and the name and title of the person administering the vaccine. All CCCs have computerized documentation of vaccine administration, and access to this information is easily available to the patient and provider. Most CCCs also participate in state registry programs where available. Participating in an immunization registry, also known as an Immunization Information System, is an efficient way to access computerized vaccine records easily at the point of contact and ensure continuity of care.

PROVIDING VACCINES IN THE CONVENIENT CARE SETTING

There are a few crucial steps the provider must conduct when a patient comes to a convenient care setting to receive a vaccine. The provider must obtain the patient's vaccine history, review with the patient or guardian the current recommendations based on age and/or health history, and third screen for contraindications to vaccine administration.

When the provider determines that a vaccine is appropriate, measures must be taken to ensure patient safety and the safe administration of the vaccine. Anyone who is to receive a vaccination, or the guardian if the person to be vaccinated is a minor, must give informed consent first. To ensure informed consent, the provider should (and, in some cases, must) provide a Vaccine Information Statement (VIS), which explains to the patient the benefits and risks of the vaccine; this gives the patient the opportunity to ask questions before consenting to receive the vaccine. The provider will then administer the vaccine following the five Rs: (1) right patient, (2) right route, (3) right dose, (4) right time, and (5) right medication.

The provider will also ensure proper documentation of the vaccine administration and provide a copy of the VIS form and the vaccine discharge instructions to the patient, reviewing normal side effects, comfort measures, and when to seek further medical attention. Patients will be instructed to wait in the clinic waiting area for at least 15 to 30 minutes after the vaccine is administered to ensure that they receive prompt intervention if they have an allergic or anaphylactic reaction to the vaccine. This is especially true in young adults, especially females, who have a greater propensity to postimmunization syncope or presyncope.

CCCs are set up for the safe administration of vaccines. All CCCs have emergency equipment to handle potential allergic reactions and anaphylaxis and should also have both adult and pediatric epinephrine and Benadryl immediately available on site. Guidelines are available regarding the administration of these medications, which are to be delivered by providers while waiting for emergency transport. Another important consideration in the safe administration of vaccines in the convenient care setting is the correct storage and temperature monitoring of vaccines. Proper storage and temperature control are crucial to providing effective and safe vaccinations. CCCs are equipped with refrigerators and have documented systems and processes in place to monitor the refrigerator temperature throughout the day and to react to potential vaccine excursions. Backup refrigerators are available to store the vaccines in the case of a temperature excursion or power outages. If a vaccine excursion does occur, the manufacturer is contacted to determine the viability of the vaccine, and appropriate actions are taken. Every clinic should have a set policy for recording the lot number and expiration date of the vaccines and a log to record the temperature of the refrigerator on a daily basis.

One clinic uses a successful technique of creating a refrigerator "planogram." A planogram is a visual depiction of the goods and products that are placed on the shelf in a retail store. This way every shelf in every retail location is the same, making the shopping experience more convenient. The same concept can be used for the refrigerator so that every clinic in a chain will have the exact same location of vaccines in the refrigerator to prevent mix-ups. Another good technique is to put a unique identifier (such as a colored sticker) on pediatric vaccinations and a label with expiration dates on the outside of all multidose vials. Finally, it is good practice to never predraw vaccinations into syringes. This practice increases the potential for errors, especially during flu season.

RESPONDING TO AN ERROR OR AN ADVERSE REACTION

When a vaccine error is made, full disclosure is always the best policy. Each clinic should have a best practice for how to report, track, and respond to vaccination errors. In addition, clinicians should be aware of mandatory reporting requirements and use of the Vaccine Adverse Event Reporting System.

In the rare instance in which a vaccination error occurs, the CDC is a great resource and they have a call line, 1-800-CDC-INFO, that can help determine the appropriate action in response to an error.

In general, clinical responses to errors include:

- If a patient receives an excessive dose, observe the patient for the usual 15-minute period. The risk of local side effects (e.g., redness, tenderness, swelling) is increased but the risk of serious side effects is not.
- If it is discovered that a patient is given too low a dose (e.g., an adult receives a pediatric dose), the remaining dose should be administered immediately. If the error is discovered after the visit, the patient should return for immunization with the correct dose.

- If a vaccine is given at the right dose but without the right indication (e.g., a vaccine not approved for pediatrics is given to a pediatric patient), the dose does not need to be repeated.
- If the patient receives an expired vaccine, the dose should be repeated from a current batch.

These are the general guidelines. For specific errors, please contact the CDC or drug manufacturer.

RESOURCES FOR HEALTH CARE PROFESSIONALS

Immunization recommendations for adults and children change rapidly. It is the individual health care provider's responsibility to be knowledgeable about the current recommendations and about individual vaccine indications and contraindications. However, to increase provider knowledge and comfort with vaccinations, clinic administration should create tools and tips for proper immunization. This can include developing inclusion and exclusion checklists for patients to use and building them into the electronic medical record. Removing any barrier for the patient or the provider can help increase immunizations, which is good for the patient, community, and business.

The CDC offers a number of helpful resources, including www.cdc.gov/vaccines/hcp.htm for providers, general information site of the Advisory Committee on Immunization Practices, www.cdc.gov/vaccines/acip/index.html, and the Immunization Action Coalition's vaccination Q & A site, www.immunize.org/askexperts.

In summary, CCCs offer a unique opportunity to promote health and prevent disease in our country by providing convenient public access to vaccines. Every encounter with a patient should include discussion of vaccination status and advocacy of needed immunizations. Only those patients presenting with more serious acute illness do not qualify for receiving a vaccination—every other patient on every visit should be asked about and offered vaccinations when appropriate. Barriers to vaccinations must be addressed and myths dispelled. It is important for the provider to know the up-to-date vaccine recommendations and true contraindications and have resources available to determine correct administration of the vaccine. With this approach, the *Healthy People 2020* vaccination targets can be achieved. Providers educated and armed with the most current information are at the forefront in ensuring that our population is adequately immunized against vaccine-preventable diseases and promoting health in our nation.

14

Making Sense of the Over-the-Counter Market

ELLIOTT M. SOGOL

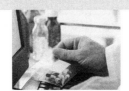

Over-the-counter (OTC) medications play an important role in managing many of the most common complaints treated in a convenient care setting. Not only do convenient care clinic (CCC) providers play a crucial role in understanding which medications are appropriate for what conditions, but they also should be familiar with what products their pharmacy carries; in addition to understanding the clinical aspects of the medications, CCC staff should routinely browse their OTC aisles to familiarize themselves with the products. Having strong relationships with the pharmacy staff and reaching out to shoppers in the OTC aisles are great ways to promote clinic awareness and promote responsible OTC use.

This chapter focuses on common OTC categories that patients use and on how convenient care clinicians can assist patients with OTC medication decisions. This chapter also describes how clinicians can work closely with pharmacists to provide patients with information to make informed decisions on appropriate OTC medication selection and use, including how to read the drug facts labels required by the Food and Drug Administration (FDA).

As the OTC market continues to grow, there are many clinically based references available for clinicians to review in more depth. The American Pharmacists Association publishes the *Handbook of Nonprescription Drugs* and recommends it as a reference for those looking for a more detailed analysis of self-care protocols and specific pharmacological and nonpharmacological interventions.

BACKGROUND

In the United States, there are two general classifications of medications: prescription (sometimes referred to as "legend" products) and nonprescription. A prescription medication is one that, because of its toxicity or potential for harm if used incorrectly, its method of use, or the collateral measures necessary for its use, has been deemed by the FDA as safe and effective for use only under the supervision of a licensed health care provider. Nonprescription, or OTC, medicines include all drugs not meeting the above definition. In general, OTC medications treat symptoms or conditions that can be self-diagnosed, can be adequately labeled for use, have a favorable benefit-risk profile when used without a provider's supervision, and have a low potential for misuse and abuse. Currently, the FDA is reviewing the possibility of creating an additional class of drug called behind-the-counter that would only be available through a pharmacist.

OTC medicines play an important role in the U.S. health care system and are important for the management of many common symptoms and conditions, including fever, mild-to-moderate pain, common cold and flu symptoms (e.g., nasal congestion, cough), allergies, heartburn, diarrhea, constipation, dermatitis, nicotine addiction, and treatment of head lice. Access to OTC products allows those with conditions amenable to self-care access to important treatment options that are efficacious, convenient, cost-effective, and generally well tolerated when used according to the label instructions.

One OTC market analysis projects that total U.S. OTC revenues will exceed $70 billion by 2015 (Visiongain, 2010). Table 14.1 provides the Consumer Healthcare Products Association's (CHPA) sales figures from 2008 to 2011 in common OTC categories, excluding herbals, vitamins, minerals, and supplements.

Table 14.1 ■ OTC Sales by Category: 2008–2011

OTC CATEGORY	2008 ($ IN MILLIONS)	2009 ($ IN MILLIONS)	2010 ($ IN MILLIONS)	2011 ($ IN MILLIONS)
Acne remedies	338	339	350	363
Analgesics, external	318	305	313	337
Analgesics, internal (includes other pain products)	2,451	2,492	2,341	2,357
Antidiarrheals	169	166	163	144
Antismoking products	493	494	485	494

OTC CATEGORY	2008 ($ IN MILLIONS)	2009 ($ IN MILLIONS)	2010 ($ IN MILLIONS)	2011 ($ IN MILLIONS)
Cough/cold and related	4,083	4,207	4,054	4,237
First aid	645	650	675	686
Foot care	349	336	336	340
Heartburn (includes antigas)	1,242	1,270	1,386	1,354
Laxatives	807	822	832	875
Oral antiseptics and rinses	744	731	722	754
All others	2,515	2,525	2,557	2,611

Source: The Nielsen Company (total U.S.—food, drug, and mass, excluding Walmart); CHPA (2012).

Figures are in millions of U.S. dollars and are approximate for 52 weeks ending the Saturday prior to January 1 of a given year. A few categories include a combination of OTC medicines and health-related products that are not classified as medicines by the FDA.

The role of the provider is to help guide the patient to make an informed choice. All medications, including OTC medications, must be taken responsibly, and the provider can assist patients and consumers in determining whether any disease state, concurrent medication, or allergies would contraindicate their choices. In addition, special considerations such as age, pregnancy, or lactation can affect the recommended OTC medications.

PATIENT INFORMATION FOR OVER-THE-COUNTER MEDICATIONS

Whenever a new medicine is prescribed or an OTC medication is recommended, it is important for providers to equip patients with appropriate instructions for use, including explaining the indication and active ingredient, dose (single and maximum daily), dosing frequency, precautions, potential side effects, duration of use, and what to do if symptoms do not improve or worsen. Much of this information is included on the labels of OTC products, but reinforcement from providers is helpful for facilitating appropriate use (National Council and Patient Information and Education [NCPIE], www.talkaboutrx.org/message.jsp). Providers must not only respond to patients' questions but also proactively supply them with relevant information. Providers are advised to confer with patients about other illnesses they have, particularly about what other prescription and OTC medications the patient is using. Other information to elicit from or share with the patient includes proper use of the intended OTC medication and its potential interactions with other medications or disease states; possible side effects; known allergies; proper dosing instructions, including how long to take the medication; and for whom the medication is intended, especially if the recipient is a child, older adult, or other dependent. It is also important to find out what OTC medications have been tried in the past—providers need to know what patients have already tried so that they do not prescribe or recommend medications that the patient already knows did not work.

In addition to the universally applicable questions identified above, certain special populations warrant more specified inquiry. For example, as noted in Chapter 12, children's dosages should be based on their weight rather than their age; thus, the provider will need to weigh the child before recommending a dosage. Providers should also clearly emphasize instructions to use the designated dosing device if one is included (e.g., medicine dosing cup; oral syringe) and be prepared to provide one, because household teaspoons and tablespoons do not provide accurate measurement. It is actually recommended that providers give recommended dosages in milliliters rather than teaspoons to discourage the use of household utensils (NCPIE, 2004).

COMMUNICATION IS THE KEY

The FDA has standardized many components of OTC medication labels for ease of patient understanding and to minimize abuse or misuse (see Figure 14.1). Patients are strongly encouraged to thoroughly read the label and to ask any questions about the information it contains.

The FDA stipulates that the following information must appear on the label and in this order (FDA, 2009):

- The product's active ingredients, including the amount in each dosage unit
- The purpose of the medication
- The uses (indications) for the medication
- Specific warnings, including when the medicine should not be used under any circumstances and when it is appropriate to consult with a doctor or pharmacist before use; this section also describes side effects that could occur and substances or activities to avoid.
- Dosage directions (who should be taking the medication, when, how, and how often)
- The product's inactive ingredients, which is helpful for avoiding ingredients that could trigger an allergic reaction

---

Drug Facts

Active ingredient (in each tablet)   **Purpose**
Chlorpheniramine maleate 2 mg .... Antihistamine

Uses temporarily relieves these symptoms due to hay fever or other upper respiratory allergies:
■ sneezing   ■ runny nose   ■ itchy, watery eyes   ■ itchy throat

---

Warnings
Ask a doctor before use if you have
■ glaucoma   ■ a breathing problem such as emphysema or chronic bronchitis
■ trouble urinating due to an enlarged prostate gland

Ask a doctor or pharmacist before use if you are taking tranquillizers or sedatives

When using this product
■ You may get drowsy   ■ avoid alcoholic drinks
■ alcohol, sedatives, and tranquillizers may increase drowsiness
■ be careful when driving a motor vehicle or operating machinery
■ excitability may occur, especially in children

If pregnant or breast-feeding, ask a health professional before use.
Keep out of reach of children. In case of overdose, get medical help or contact a Poison Control
Center right away.

Directions

adults and children 12 years and over	take 2 tablets every 4 to 6 hours; not more than 12 tablets in 24 hours
children 6 years to under 12 years	take 1 tablet every 4 to 6 hours; not more than 6 tablets in 24 hours
children under 6 years	ask a doctor

Other information store at 20–25° C (68–77° F)   ■ protect from excessive moisture

---

Inactive ingredients D&C yellow no. 10, lactose, magnesium stearate, microcrystalline
cellulose, pregelatinized starch

Figure 14.1 ■ Food and Drug Administration sample drug facts label (FDA, 2009).

COUGH AND COLD

As noted in Table 14.1, cough and cold products lead the way in OTC purchases, with over $4.2 billion in sales for 2011. Consumers use these products to treat the symptoms of cough, runny nose, stuffy nose, congestion, sinus drip, and myriad other symptoms. The FDA has limited the use of some of these products for children younger than 4 years, and they are no longer recommended. In addition, some patients will ask about herbal remedies or so-called megadoses of certain vitamins, but there is little evidence in the literature to support their use or indicate that they are curative. Humidifiers can also be helpful, particularly in the fall and winter when heaters are running and indoor air is drier. The added moisture in the air can help relieve itchy eyes and throat, cracked lips, and dry skin.

Common Cold

The common cold is usually a mild, self-limiting illness, primarily caused by the rhinovirus. It is estimated that Americans suffer from more than 1 billion colds each year (National Center for Complementary and Alternative Medicine, 2012). The goal in treating a patient with a cold is to help alleviate or control symptoms, typically runny nose, congestion, coughing, itchy or sore throat, body aches or headaches, and others. Recommendations for OTC medications should be aimed at relieving the patient's most problematic symptoms: decongestants and saline nasal sprays can relieve congestion and antihistamines, alone or combined with a decongestant, can treat the runny nose. Patients with a number of cold symptoms may benefit from a combination product, but there is a risk with these products of multipharmacy side effects because these products contain a mixture of different medications. In addition, many combination products contain the same ingredients regardless of the condition they claim to treat (common cold, cold and flu, cough and cold, sinus headache, etc.); the most prevalent combination seems to be a first-generation antihistamine with a nasal decongestant. Thus, clinicians must educate patients about these products' ingredients to ensure that patients are not taking multiple products with the same ingredients and decrease the risk of overdose on a given medication.

For nasal decongestion, pseudoephedrine is the strongest available OTC medication, although it is now sold behind the pharmacy counter and patients must present identification or other documentation to purchase it. Phenylephrine is an alternative decongestant that can be purchased straight from the shelf. Antihistamines primarily vary by sedative effect; first-generation products (diphenhydramine, brompheniramine, chlorpheniramine, and clemastine) tend to make users sleepy, and some patients may prefer or require the limited sedative effectives of second- or third-generation antihistamines (loratadine, cetirizine, fexofenadine).

As is the case with many prescription medications, OTC medications should be used with caution in pregnant and lactating women; providers must weigh the benefits against the risks of all medications. Again, single-ingredient products reduce the multipharmacy side effects of combination products.

Nasal sprays (saline, ephedrine, naphazoline, oxymetazoline, phenylephrine) can be recommended. However, medicated sprays should be used for only up to 3 days, or the patient runs the risk of nasal rebound congestion. Saline sprays can be used for longer if necessary.

Cough

Cough can be attributed to a variety of underlying causes including viral infections, bacterial infections, asthma, and smoking. In addition, cough can be caused by some medications (some angiotensin-converting-enzyme inhibitors are the most common). Because of the range of potential origins of a cough, treatment with an OTC medication should be specific to those conditions that are self-limiting. In addition, different OTC medications will be applicable depending on the symptomatology of the cough (i.e., productive or dry and nonproductive).

As with the common cold, providers' lines of questioning may help to determine what OTC medication will best treat a cough (see Table 14.1), assuming that OTC self-care is appropriate:

- Describe your cough.
- How bothersome is the cough?
- Does the cough keep you up at night?
- Does anything specific make the cough worse or better?
- When did the cough start?
- What have you tried for relief of your cough?
- What prescription or nonprescription medications have you taken or are currently taking?
- What medical conditions do you have?
- Do you have any medication allergies?

It should be noted that the most common OTC treatments for cough and cold, particularly pseudoephedrine and dextromethorphan, are among the most frequently abused and misused OTC medications. Providers should always recommend these products with care and an understanding of their potential for abuse.

DERMATOLOGY

Patients present to CCCs every day seeking advice and treatment for ailments that affect the skin, hair, and nails. The skin is the largest organ of the human body and provides important functions, including protection from external insults and microorganisms, temperature modulation, and synthesis of vitamin D.

Topical medications for skin ailments can come as ointments, creams, lotions, or gels. Table 14.2 can help a provider decide when to use which.

ANALGESICS

Pain has been reported as one of the primary reasons patients seek medical care, and it is very subjective (American Academy of Pain Management, n.d.; Berardi, 2009; Loeser & Melzack, 1999).

Patients seek advice for OTC medications for any number of conditions including sprains, strains, contusions, muscle soreness, tendinitis, and arthritis among many others, giving the CCC provider the opportunity to educate patients about OTC options and make appropriate choices. Providers can and should also underscore the importance of both pharmacologic and nonpharmacologic treatments. For acute nonserious musculoskeletal injuries,

Table 14.2 ■ **Dosage Forms for Topical Therapy (Emollients and Corticosteroids)**

DOSAGE FORM	ADVANTAGES	DISADVANTAGES
Ointment	Provides maximal lubrication and occlusion Useful for dry and thick lesions Improves penetration of other agents	Thick, greasy Not preferred for hairy areas
Cream	Vanishes quickly into skin Lubricating/moisturizing Drying effect for weepy lesions	Less potent compared with ointments Minimally occlusive Often contains preservatives, which may cause irritation
Lotion/gel	Least greasy, with minimal residue Drying effect for weepy lesions Useful for hairy areas of skin	Least occlusive Less potent compared with ointments

Source: Ference and Last (2009).

nonpharmacotherapy treatment typically begins with the standard RICE therapy (rest, ice, compression, and elevation): "Rest Injury for 1 to 2 days, Ice for 10 to 15 minutes three or four times a day for 1 to 2 days (or longer for severe injuries), apply Compress with elastic supports being sure that the support is not too tight to decrease circulation, and finally Elevate the injury above the heart if possible" (National Institute of Arthritis, Musculoskeletal and Skin Diseases, 2009).

Pharmacotherapy for mild-to-moderate pain usually includes acetaminophen, nonsteroidal anti-inflammatory drugs (NSAIDs) such as aspirin, naproxen sodium, and ibuprofen, or external (topical) analgesics such as camphor, phenol, capsaicin, and others. Because of the subjective nature of pain and its treatment, a regimented approach provides patients with the understanding that they should treat for a day or two to keep the pain in check.

The potential for overusing and exceeding the daily dosage limits of OTC medications must be reviewed with the patient, especially with any type of acetaminophen. To help encourage appropriate acetaminophen use and reduce the risk of accidental overdose, new dosing guidelines and label instructions have been issued that lower the maximum daily dose of some single-ingredient acetaminophen-containing products sold in the United States from 4,000 to 3,000 mg.

In addition, providers should ensure that patients are not already taking any acetaminophen-containing products such as combination OTC products or prescription analgesics. Many patients may not realize that a number of prescription analgesics are combination products that contain acetaminophen, and they can easily exceed the maximum daily dose by concurrently using OTC acetaminophen. Finally, patients should be counseled regarding concomitant use of alcohol with acetaminophen and the risk of liver toxicity over long-term use.

Aspirin and NSAIDs also bring a measure of concern because of the potential for gastrointestinal upset or bleeding. Providers should counsel patients on potential symptoms related to these side effects and emphasize the benefit of taking the medications with food.

Finally, topical preparations generally work as counterirritants, stimulating pain receptors. A concern with these OTC medications is primarily irritation at the site of application.

CONCLUSION

For patients to make safe OTC medication choices, they must be armed with the knowledge of what are appropriate conditions for self-care and what are appropriate treatment choices. Thus, providers must understand the clinical indications and side effects of the various OTC products. Practitioners in retail locations that have a pharmacy should familiarize themselves with the OTC selections available at their stores' pharmacies. Spending time in the pharmacy OTC area is a great technique to get familiar with the products and to interact with shoppers and build a relationship with them. If time permits, walking a patient into the OTC aisle to help them choose the appropriate product is a great way to create a fantastic patient experience.

15

Strategies to Improve Antibiotic Prescribing in Convenient Care

REBECCA M. ROBERTS, LAURI A. HICKS, AND JOSHUA RIFF

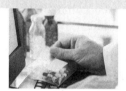

Antibiotic resistance is one of the world's most pressing health threats, and antibiotic use is the primary contributor to this growing issue (Harrison & Lederberg, 1998). A study in the late 1990s revealed that antibiotics were prescribed in 68% of acute respiratory tract visits and that, of those, almost 80% were unnecessary according to Centers for Disease Control and Prevention (CDC) guidelines (Scott et al., 2001). Antibiotic overprescribing contributes not only to bacterial antibiotic resistance but also to poor patient outcomes in terms of complications and adverse drug events (Shehab, Patel, Srinivasan, & Budnitz, 2008). Antibiotic-resistant infections are more challenging and costly to treat and are associated with increased patient mortality. A study evaluating the association between antibiotic prescribing and nonsusceptibility among invasive pneumococcal disease isolates found that in areas where antibiotic prescribing was high, incidence of nonsusceptible pneumococcal disease was also high, indicating that local prescribing practices contribute to local resistance patterns (Hicks, Chien, Taylor, Haber, & Klugman, 2011). The prescribing behaviors of providers in all settings—including convenient care clinics (CCCs)—are critical in ensuring that antibiotics are being prescribed only when necessary and at the appropriate dose and duration for each diagnosis.

CONVENIENT CARE MEDICINE AND APPROPRIATE ANTIBIOTIC USE

With the rapid emergence of and expansion in the number of CCCs in the United States, it is important to take a closer look at prescribing and to provide support to those practicing in this setting, especially because the common conditions (e.g., upper respiratory infections [URIs]) seen in retail-based clinics are also the conditions for which antibiotics are inappropriately prescribed (Mehrotra et al., 2009). One common perception of the general public and the medical community is that CCCs and their co-located pharmacies are good places for self-diagnosed patients to easily receive medications including antibiotics. However, one study among enrollees in a large Minnesota health plan has shown that antibiotic prescribing in retail clinics does not differ from prescribing in traditional provider offices (Mehrotra et al., 2009). In addition, a 2011 quality measurement report issued by Minnesota Community Measurement based on health plan claims showed that two retail clinic providers in Minnesota were less likely to prescribe an antibiotic for adults with a diagnosis of bronchitis when compared with all medical groups in the state that reported data (MN Community Measurement, 2010). Although these studies and measures are specific to Minnesota (where CCCs originated and are quite common), they suggest that antibiotic use in adults for bronchitis in retail clinics may be comparable with or even better than its use in traditional primary care provider office settings. Recent antibiotic prescribing data for children indicate that 58% of all antibiotic prescriptions written in the outpatient setting are for URIs that are predominantly viral in nature (Grijalva, Nuorti, & Griffin, 2009; Centers for Disease Control, 2011). One potential reason for this is that providers have limited time to counsel patients and often mistakenly assume that a patient presenting with such an infection expects an antibiotic (Stivers, Mangione-Smith, Elliott, McDonald, & Heritage, 2003). The outpatient setting accounts for more than 60% of antibiotic expenditures in the United States (Hicks, 2010), and with the number of CCCs increasing steadily (Mehrotra et al., 2009), efforts to characterize antibiotic prescribing in retail clinics and support appropriate antibiotic prescribing practices are critical. It is incumbent on providers and management to establish practices, policies, and procedures that promote safe, appropriate, and effective prescribing.

STRATEGIES TO ENCOURAGE APPROPRIATE ANTIBIOTIC PRESCRIBING

There are a number of strategies that convenient care clinic management and providers can adopt to reduce inappropriate antibiotic prescribing.

Strategies for Providers

There are several strategies that can improve patient satisfaction and enhance provider knowledge and prescribing performance. Studies have revealed that providers overestimate the frequency that patients and parents expect to receive an antibiotic prescription. In one study, pediatricians prescribed antibiotics 62%

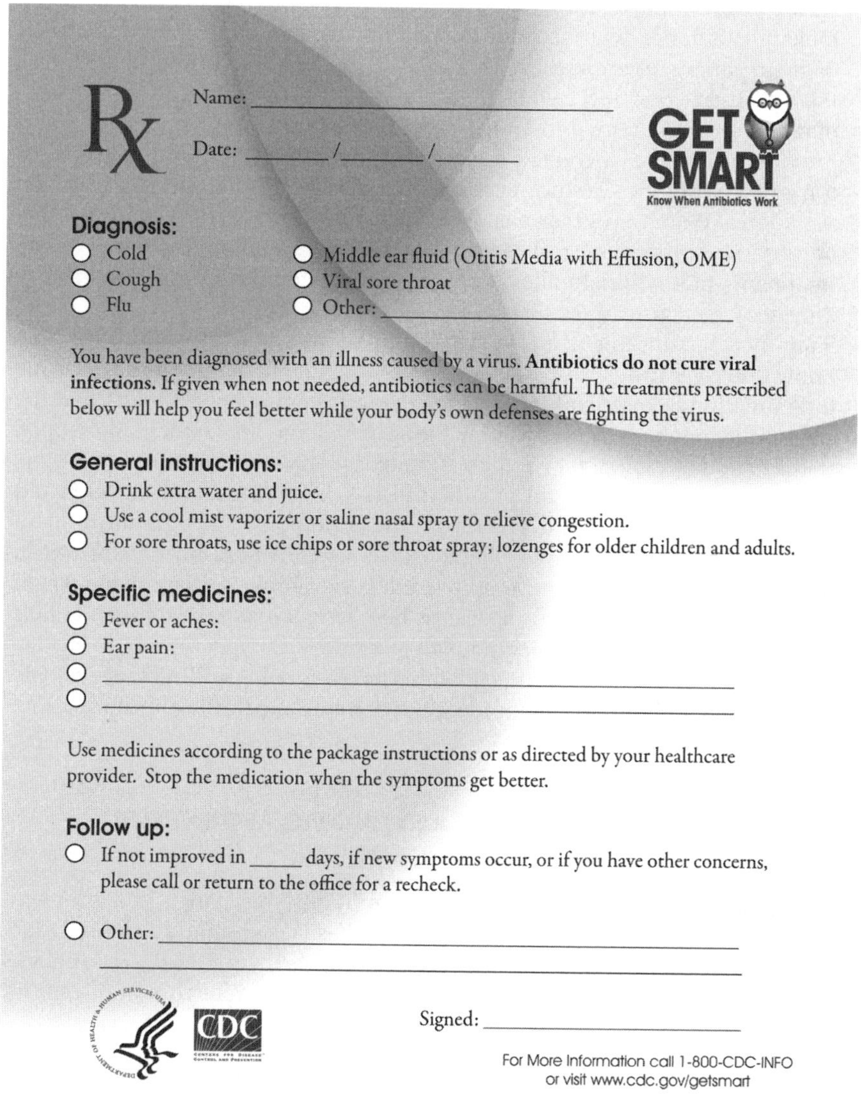

℞ Name: ____________________

Date: ______/______/______

GET SMART
Know When Antibiotics Work

Diagnosis:

- O Cold
- O Cough
- O Flu
- O Middle ear fluid (Otitis Media with Effusion, OME)
- O Viral sore throat
- O Other: ____________________

You have been diagnosed with an illness caused by a virus. **Antibiotics do not cure viral infections.** If given when not needed, antibiotics can be harmful. The treatments prescribed below will help you feel better while your body's own defenses are fighting the virus.

General instructions:

- O Drink extra water and juice.
- O Use a cool mist vaporizer or saline nasal spray to relieve congestion.
- O For sore throats, use ice chips or sore throat spray; lozenges for older children and adults.

Specific medicines:

- O Fever or aches:
- O Ear pain:
- O ____________________
- O ____________________

Use medicines according to the package instructions or as directed by your healthcare provider. Stop the medication when the symptoms get better.

Follow up:

- O If not improved in _____ days, if new symptoms occur, or if you have other concerns, please call or return to the office for a recheck.
- O Other: ____________________

Signed: ____________________

CDC

For More Information call 1-800-CDC-INFO or visit www.cdc.gov/getsmart

Figure 15.1 ■ Get Smart: Know When Antibiotics Work viral prescription pad.

of the time if they perceived parents expected a prescription compared with 7% of the time if they did not feel parents expected a prescription, highlighting the importance of having an open discussion with patients about this issue (Mangione-Smith et al., 2004). When an antibiotic is not indicated, here are recommended strategies to improve patient and parent satisfaction:

- Provide a specific diagnosis to help patients feel validated. For example, say "viral bronchitis" instead of referring to an illness as "just a virus."
- Provide clear instructions and recommend symptomatic relief. This can make a difference when a patient does not require an antibiotic. Patients or their parents often request an antibiotic because they think it will help them or their child feel better; they may not realize that effective symptomatic therapies can give them the relief they are seeking. Some clinics and provider offices have created patient handouts and discharge instructions for when antibiotics are not needed. The CDC's "Get Smart: Know When Antibiotics Work" program has developed a viral prescription pad that can be used to "prescribe" rest, specific symptomatic relief, and other home treatments that will help alleviate symptoms of common upper respiratory illnesses (see Figure 15.1).
- Share normal findings during the examination. For example, let patients know that their lungs sound clear or reassure parents that there is no visible inflammation in their child's ear. This reassures patients or parents that the illness may not be as severe as they thought and may make them more open to the idea that they don't need an antibiotic.
- Discuss potential side effects of antibiotic use, including adverse events and resistance. Many patients don't realize that antibiotics can be harmful.
- Explain to patients or parents what to expect over the next few days. This can help them feel reassured and empowered. For example, explain that a cough may persist for several days, or discuss how long it may take for their child's earache to subside. Give patients a plan of action in case symptoms do change or become more severe, and note that this includes being willing to reevaluate the situation and prescribe antibiotics if it becomes medically appropriate.

CLINICAL PEARLS FOR ANTIBIOTIC AVOIDANCE

Although most providers are aware that antibiotic resistance is a problem largely created by antibiotic overuse, research has shown that this knowledge alone is insufficient to change provider practice (Schwartz, Bell, & Hughes, 1997). Criteria to determine when antibiotics are indicated for common respiratory infections can be found in Table 15.1.

Acute bronchitis (Gonzales et al., 2001): Acute bronchitis is a common syndrome with a chief complaint of cough. It is caused by a virus in more than 90% of cases, and there are no indications for prescribing antibiotics for patients who are not immunocompromised (Chapman, Henderson, Clyde, Collier, & Denny, 1981). The most important feature when diagnosing bronchitis

Table 15.1 ■ Criteria to Determine When Antibiotics Are Indicated for Common Respiratory Infections

	ACUTE PHARYNGITIS	ACUTE OTITIS MEDIA	ACUTE SINUSITIS	ACUTE BRONCHITIS	NONSPECIFIC UPPER RESPIRATORY INFECTION (COMMON COLD)
Suspect bacterial infection *if*	At least two of the following: fever, tonsillar exudates, tender lymph nodes, absent cough	Middle-ear effusion plus signs of inflammation	Persistent, severe, or worsening symptoms	Acute cough, new focal chest signs, shortness of breath, tachypnea, and a fever; rule out pneumonia	Not bacterial
Initiate antibiotic treatment *if*	Clinical diagnosis plus positive strep test	Otalgia and middle ear effusion plus* 1. Moderate to severe bulging, redness 2. Otorrhea in absence of otitis externa	1. More than 10 days of purulent rhinorrhea without clinical improvement 2. High fever (>39°C/102°F), purulent nasal discharge, facial pain 3. Worsening symptoms despite initial improvement (double sickening)	Antibiotics are rarely indicated for acute bronchitis	Antibiotics are never indicated for the common cold

Note: *Observation or watchful waiting is appropriate in some cases of children ≥6 months of age.

is to rule out pneumonia. Patients with an acute cough and new focal chest signs, shortness of breath, tachypnea, and a fever should be suspected of having pneumonia. It is important to note that green sputum production can occur whether the infection is bacterial or viral and does not help to determine whether an antibiotic is needed.

Nonspecific upper respiratory tract infection and common cold (Gonzales et al., 2001): All colds are caused by viral infections. Despite misconceptions, a cold can last up to 14 days, and green purulent nasal secretions do not make a bacterial infection more likely (Arruda, Pitkaranta, Witek, Doyle, & Hayden, 1997). The common cold is self-limited, and antibiotics should never be prescribed for its treatment.

Acute pharyngitis (Shulman et al., 2012): Pharyngitis, or sore throat, may be accompanied by other nonspecific symptoms including cough, congestion, and fever. A critical diagnostic consideration is whether Group A streptococcus (GAS) is the cause. Unlike acute otitis media (AOM) and acute bacterial sinusitis, the diagnosis of GAS requires utilization of a confirmatory laboratory test. Patients should only be tested for GAS if they meet specific clinical criteria, and antibiotic treatment is only indicated if the test result is positive.

Acute sinusitis (Chow et al., 2012): In general, most cases of sinusitis are due to uncomplicated viral infections. Bacterial sinusitis should be considered when symptoms have been present for greater than 10 days without improvement, symptoms are severe, or the patient has worsening symptoms after initial improvement from a URI (double sickening).

Acute otitis media: AOM may be defined as the rapid onset of signs and symptoms of inflammation in the middle ear. These include bulging and/or erythema of the tympanic membrane (TM) and symptoms such as irritability, ottorrhea, otalgia, and fever. The diagnosis of AOM always requires a careful examination with an otoscope to confirm the presence of an inflamed TM. Although clear visualization of the TM can be difficult, a high degree of diagnostic certainty is needed to avoid antibiotic overuse. In addition, in patients aged 6 months or older and meeting certain criteria, an "observation option" or "watchful waiting period" can be followed, provided that the patient is able to return for a follow-up visit if symptoms do not resolve on their own or worsen (Subcommittee on Management of Acute Otitis Media, 2004).

STRATEGIES FOR CONVENIENT CARE CLINIC MANAGEMENT

Educate providers and patients: There are many existing resources that can be used for provider and patient education. The CDC's "Get Smart: Know When Antibiotics Work" program offers free educational materials in print and online for both providers and patients. This program aims to reduce the rate of increase of antibiotic resistance by:

- Promoting adherence to appropriate prescribing guidelines among providers

- Decreasing demand for antibiotics for viral URIs among healthy adults and parents of young children
- Increasing adherence to prescribed antibiotics for URIs
- Download resources or order print materials from the Get Smart website: www.cdc.gov/getsmart.

Gather and use data for provider feedback: One of the more effective techniques CCC leadership can employ is monthly or quarterly reporting that ranks providers on antibiotic prescribing for conditions such as bronchitis or URIs. The more transparent this ranking is at the provider level, the more likely the program will be effective. Such data collection can also be used to target specific providers or clinics for additional education.

Utilize technology: Using prompts built into the electronic health record, otherwise known as clinical decision support, is one way to assist providers. Clinical decision support can be used to determine whether an antibiotic is needed, guide symptomatic therapy, and promote selection of the correct antibiotic and dose if one is needed. If electronic clinical decision support is not feasible, paper-based clinical decision support also has been shown to be effective.

THE FUTURE

A multifaceted approach is needed to minimize the impact of antibiotic resistance on our future. Prevention of infections, through optimization of vaccination programs and infection prevention strategies, is one approach. Providers also need access to reliable and rapid diagnostics that can inform treatment decisions. Finally, all providers need to practice antibiotic stewardship; this means prescribing only when an antibiotic is indicated and prescribing the appropriate drug, dose, and duration for the diagnosis. Promoting and practicing appropriate antibiotic use are essential components of efforts to reduce the spread of antibiotic resistance, and the convenient care industry can and should be a leader in this effort.

16

Building and Marketing a Retail Clinic

MARY KATE SCOTT

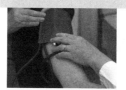

As noted in Chapter 2, interest in the convenient care industry (CCI) has expanded as convenient care clinics (CCCs) have demonstrated that they have a role to fill in the health care industry. They provide comparable (when not superior) care to that of the mainstream industry at affordable prices. And, most importantly, they are convenient. Their extended operating hours, locations within large retailers, and defined scopes of service appeal to customers in a variety of ways: CCCs serve patients who cannot get to their primary care doctors during regular business hours, or who do not have regular doctors; the limited services they provide allow for quick handling of straightforward ailments that don't require extensive treatment; and they serve as one more errand retail shoppers can accomplish all in one location. Although freestanding retail-based clinics that offer limited, specific scopes of service and expanded hours are CCCs, this book's focus is on clinics that are or will be located within retail settings.

Given the attractive qualities that CCCs present consumers, retailers are keen to learn more about CCCs and how they benefit their strategies and customers. They are interested to understand whether these clinics can bring in new customers or increase revenue, or improve their reputation within the community. Similarly, clinic operators are interested to understand how CCCs could improve profitability. Basing a clinic within a retail location could bring an operator into a new neighborhood in a cost-effective way and bring the retailer added business as well.

CCCs can be an attractive proposition for both retailers and clinic operators, but there are many factors that have to be carefully addressed if the relationship is to be profitable for both parties. Usually it is an existing clinic operator who wants to explore new locations, so the onus is on the operator to conduct necessary research to make a compelling case to a prospective retailer. The clinic operator needs to identify a suitable retail partner; establish an optimal location; determine the most appropriate scope of services; and assess the impact of a new location on existing operations. If there is insufficient market demand, or the location does not offer new customers, a new CCC may not be suitable.

SELECTING A RETAIL PARTNER

After the decision to consider a convenient care clinic, the clinic operator must select a retail partner. Operators need to understand retailers' reputations, offerings, store locations, and customer base. Greater familiarity with the retailer improves an operator's chances of success when presenting the proposal.

Most retailers are part of national chains, but many, especially drug and grocery stores, operate independently or are part of regional or local chains. The clinic operator needs to identify which retailers might be open to CCCs. As discussed in Chapter 2, a number of national retailers entered the retail-based clinic industry in the mid-2000s, including CVS Caremark, Walgreens, and Kroger; these retailers own and operate their own CCCs, so operators are unlikely to secure space for new clinics within any of these stores' locations. A number of merchants, including Walmart, Rite Aid, and Albertsons, have relationships with multiple CCC operators, enabling them to select those with expertise and experience appropriate for a particular community. Retailers with existing CCC relationships are more likely to be open to new clinics at their stores.

Location

Operators should be prepared to present to the retailer financial estimates of the leasing fees and increased customer revenue an in-store CCC could be expected to generate. Once economic arrangements are in place, the retailer and clinic operator will need to determine which store location will be the best fit. The two most important factors to look for are support from in-store management and a sufficient number of appropriate shoppers. Consumer visits to the retailer are critical: For a clinic to be viable, a drugstore should receive at least 8,000 weekly shopper visits, a grocery store 20,000, and mass merchandisers 40,000 or more.

Another key part of the retailer decision is whether the clinic will carry the operator's brand, the retailer's, or both. Some retailers (e.g., Walmart) require that all clinics have both brands, while other retailers mandate that the clinic will carry only the operator's name. If the retailer does not have a preference, the clinic operator will need to decide what is in the best interests of the operation.

A co-branded clinic can be simpler and more cost-effective, but in exchange, the operator may have to make compromises on design, signage, and perhaps some aspects of managing the clinic. Walmart's CCC design, for example, contains specifications for layout, including the waiting area, the reception desk, and signage. Some co-branding arrangements specify that the retailer be responsible for selecting the contractor and monitoring the building process while other retailers may provide only building plans.

As part of the clinic's branding, signage is also a critical decision that retailer and operator will need to confirm in the lease; this can be a point of contention. Signage locations, size, and content can be difficult to negotiate. Considerations include the clinic's brand name and how, from patients' perspectives, the clinic is related to the operator's other locations. For example, health systems opening CCCs need to account for how signage and marketing will differentiate their retail clinics from urgent care or other walk-in care so that patients understand the services being offered. Although retailers may have certain specifications, any signage must make clear the clinic operator's involvement in the clinic; that is, the signage must make clear to the customer who the clinic's operator is, even if signs also contain the retailer's name, logo, or other form of identification.

Sign location must also be resolved. Ideally, signs should be in a number of places: on the building itself, on the front door of the clinic (if it is enclosed rather than open to the store), and on inside walls and stanchions. Retailers' requirements and preferences differ, however, so clinic operators need to be clear about what they need but also flexible enough to accommodate retailer requirements.

Negotiating the Lease

Retailers often draft the lease because they typically have in-house legal departments or they work with local counsel that specializes in commercial leasing. Nevertheless, clinic operators should play an active role in negotiating lease terms and should seek their own legal counsel. Clinic operators should keep in mind that it may take time to establish a good relationship with the retail partner and formulate an appropriate lease agreement. However, investing the time to create this solid foundation is easier than trying to exit a lease if either party's expectations are not met.

A CCC lease should include specifics about the cost of space, which should be based on fair market value as assessed by an appraiser, and should describe signage allowances and each party's responsibilities related to marketing. The lease should also specify the timing of construction, securing of permits, and the days and hours the convenient care clinic will be open. It is advised that the lease term be at least 3 years with an option to renew automatically, and counsel for both parties should be knowledgeable about any relevant local or state laws that could arise.

Design and Construction

CCCs can be as small as a single, 140-square-foot room or as large as 680 square feet with several examination rooms and a waiting area. Examination rooms must be at least 100 square feet to accommodate equipment and practitioners. Thus, a clinic with two examination rooms, corridors, a restroom, and a common area for equipment and supplies can easily occupy 400 square feet. Note that operators will also need to meet Americans with Disabilities Act (ADA) standards and requirements.

Specific factors to address in mapping out the physical space of the clinic include (but are certainly not limited to):

- Will the clinic—reception and waiting area, examination rooms, staff-only areas—be open to the store or enclosed behind walls and a door?
  - Is there sufficient space to ensure privacy during patient check-in?
  - Will there be a self-service automated check-in kiosk or will a registration/reception desk be required?
- What range of services will the clinic provide? This will determine the amount of space and associated equipment required, in particular, the number of examination rooms.
- Will the clinic have its own restroom for patients or will the clinic and the store share the main restrooms? Facilities where drug screening will be conducted have specific requirements that must be met including state regulations for proper collection.
- What type of security will be used at the clinic and who will be responsible for maintaining it (e.g., if the clinic will be open to the store, what safeguards will there be for locking up front-desk and back-office computers, examination rooms and equipment, supply closets)?

Many clinic operators work with local contractors who provide basic design services, while others engage architectural firms. Retailers who have specific templates that must be followed may also have designated contractors who are already approved to do their build-outs; in cases like that, the clinic operator will not have much say in the final design. Where the operator makes the decision, however, the choice of contractor depends on a number of factors including the operator's available resources, the complexity of the available space (e.g., awkward layout or location within the store), and the clinic's scope of service.

Regarding timing, turnaround time for construction and permits can be as fast as 8 to 10 weeks or as slow as 18 to 24 months. Where possible, operators should select local contractors who have worked in small spaces, preferably in retail settings, and are familiar with the permit process. Clinic construction also differs from other types of retail construction, so it is preferable to work with contractors who understand the particular needs of health care settings. Whoever has hired the contractor—whether clinic operator or retailer—should work closely with the contractor to ensure that construction is timely and within budget and that all permitting requirements are being met at every level.

The service menu and fee schedule should be designed so that the information is clearly displayed and may be easily changed. Many retail clinics also prominently display the operators' names and photographs and also the clinic's mission.

CLINIC OPERATIONS

Most of the retailer and operator staff working on a new clinic location typically have very little involvement in the construction. Staff who are not directly involved in monitoring clinic construction use this time to develop the operations and logistics of managing the new clinic, including marketing. By the time construction begins, the clinic's scope of service should have been established, and all necessary staff should have been identified and trained and marketing plans in place.

Staffing and Training

As discussed in Chapter 2, since their inception CCCs have been primarily staffed by nurse practitioners with support from physician assistants, and some have medical assistants as well; some may also have supervising physicians. Before the clinic opens for service, all staff need to be familiar with the clinic's scope of services, clinical protocols, patient documentation, payment processing, IT and equipment, and all other aspects of the logistics of running the clinic day to day.

A primary feature of the convenient care model is the use of electronic health records (EHRs), and many retail-based clinics use EHRs to ensure seamless and secure communication of patient data between all relevant providers (emergency departments, primary care providers, the operator's other sites, etc.). If a clinic intends to use paper charts, it must establish procedures to ensure that the right information and chart are at the right location when these are needed for patient care, quality review, or other purposes. Documentation processes need to be created for the CCC staff to ensure a streamlined intake process and copayment determination.

Quality of Care

The critical challenge of the CCI has always been demonstrating that CCCs can deliver the same quality of care as mainstream health care. However, CCCs have risen to the challenge, and, as with all other health care services, these clinics recognize that implementing quality assurance and improvement systems is critical. Thus, any clinic operators looking into opening a CCC must develop and become familiar with appropriate quality-of-care protocols and have them in place before the clinic opens. Clinic operations leadership and staff need to be prepared to take a number of steps to ensure care quality including:

- Establish standards for any primary care physicians who will oversee the clinic; standards should specify their supervision, collaboration, and chart review responsibilities
- Evaluate storage needs (i.e., equipment, medications, vaccines)
- Create incident reporting and tracking guidelines, including procedures for reporting relevant incidents to the operator's public health authorities and the retail store manager

Operators might also consider tracking patient data and trends, which could help improve quality of care and also generate valuable information for public health authorities. This information could include the most common reasons for patient visits and patients' perception of care quality.

CLINIC MARKETING

As noted earlier, the construction phase of a convenient care clinic is when many operators begin intensive marketing for the new clinic. However, many CCC operators have found marketing to be a greater challenge than they anticipated. A number of hospitals and health care systems have said that before their CCCs opened, they did not have to consider how to attract patients or how to explain a limited-service offering.

Focus on Multiple Target Audiences

Essentially, anyone who ever needs health care services is a potential customer of a convenient care clinic. However, marketing plans need to address several audiences. The target audience could be broken into a number of groups, including store customers, who are the potential patients; store personnel, who can spread the word to customers; the local medical community, who can recommend CCCs as reliable after-hours alternatives to emergency rooms; and employers. These audiences will serve different promotional purposes, so the marketing messages to each will vary. No matter the audience, however, the overall marketing challenge is to communicate:

- The benefit to the community of the new clinic, particularly the convenience of walk-in care
- The clinic's services and costs
- The accepted payment methods, including insurance
- The population the clinic will serve
- Assurance that the clinic will deliver quality care
- Connections to a medical home through the operator's other site(s), if applicable

Another challenge is limiting the marketing focus to potential patients, who may be only 2 to 5 miles away in urban settings, or farther away depending on service area and the distance local consumers commute and drive. This generally small geographic area warrants marketing via micro media, such as local newspapers and radio stations, school and place of worship newsletters, and community websites and email.

The medical community: Local health care providers make excellent target audiences for a CCC's marketing efforts. All types of medical professionals and community leaders are key sources of information for potential convenient care clinic patients. Local doctors, dentists, and other specialists can be invited to tour the clinic when it opens, either individually or through an open house. Their first-person impressions and recommendations will encourage potential patients' confidence in the clinic. Local emergency rooms may also be willing to provide brochures or postcards advertising the new CCC as an alternative for nonemergency, after-hours care.

Store personnel: Because everyone inside a store, whether staff or customers, is a potential clinic customer, it is critical that staff at the clinic's location be fully versed in the clinic's services, offerings, prices, and so forth. Along with making written materials available, managers, floor staff, pharmacy personnel, cashiers, and stockers should be prepared to promote the clinic and answer customer questions. The clinic operator takes the lead on educating staff, with the cooperation of store management. Existing retailer staff might attend informational sessions where they learn about the new clinic, and information about the clinic might be included in training for all new staff. Once the clinic is open, staff should also be encouraged to use the services.

Other operator locations: Where a new CCC is part of an existing clinic chain, the staff at existing clinic sites should also be prepared to communicate the opening of a new clinic to current patients. Brochures, posters, and other materials should be available, but staff who already work for the clinic will be in the best position to assure patients that they will obtain the same level of care at the new location. Staff at existing locations should emphasize that care will be the same but also highlight the differences and benefits of the new clinic; in many cases, this will include evening and weekend hours when the main clinic sites are closed, and guaranteed 15- to 20-minute visits. Successful CCC operators invest time with providers and staff and ensure that information about the new site is widely available to both staff and customers. Brochures and posters around the clinic (in different languages where applicable) highlighting on the clinic's website, staff informational sessions, and postcards for distribution at nearby businesses are all ways that clinic operators can notify existing customers and neighbors of the new site's location that a new convenient care clinic will be opening.

Existing clinic and store customers: Current clinic customers make an excellent source of referral visits to a new convenient care clinic. Consider e-mail and paper mailings to existing customers to let them know of the new clinic including its hours and services.

Store promotions can also include advertisements for the new clinic. Ongoing in-store marketing might include alerting customers on when flu shots will be available, offering back-to-school vaccination and physical examination specials, and highlighting clinic hours.

The opening of a new CCC is an exciting and newsworthy event. Operators should aim for the official grand opening to be 2 to 3 weeks after the clinic has started seeing its first patients. This brief period allows clinic staff to become comfortable with the new site—new routines, equipment, procedures, and so forth—and to work out kinks before opening for widespread business. This pregrand opening period might be a good time to offer store employees discounts, or even free visits, to ensure awareness.

The grand opening also makes an ideal venue for inviting local media. Clinic leadership should be prepared to share how the new CCC will benefit the community and address its health care needs and how it fits within the spectrum of the operator's services. Patient testimonials about service at the clinic can also help boost community confidence in the new clinic. And many retailers are willing to help by providing a public relations toolkit, press releases, and contacts.

EVALUATION, OPERATIONAL MEASURES, AND QUALITY OF CARE

Many convenient care clinic operators assess the success of their new clinic based on operational measures including daily, weekly, and monthly patient volume; number of patients who return and who report that they intend to return; and patient satisfaction with services. These measures shed light on which marketing programs work, including which advertisements and campaigns generated patient traffic and which events brought in new or existing patients. Clinic operators also conduct "mystery shopper visits" to evaluate their clinics regarding service quality, greeting, wait time, cleanliness, and the availability of information to consumers. Some send surveys to or interview store managers to assess the quality of the clinic–store relationship.

Operators are also likely to be interested in how well the clinic delivers on its goals while delivering quality care, enhancing provider satisfaction, ensuring operational excellence, and meeting financial goals. In particular, the new clinic's financial impact on overall clinic operations and the store is likely to be of interest to clinic leadership.

Patient and Provider Satisfaction

Quality-of-care measures are paramount for any health care service; retail-based health care has a vested interest in demonstrating that high-quality, affordable health care can be delivered without the requirements and restrictions of traditional care. For clinic operators, critical components to track include provider adherence to evidence-based guidelines and patient histories and compliance with any physician oversight requirements (such as local or state regulations or clinic peer review measures).

Many clinics monitor the frequency of patients who present with conditions that can't be best treated at the convenient care clinic level, particularly whether these patients seek services at other sites within the operator's care network or elsewhere entirely. Tracking of the frequency of certain conditions and their outcomes can also give operators an idea of where their resources might best be focused and where they need improvement.

Most if not all CCCs track patient satisfaction, generally through surveys. In many cases, the provider contacts patients 48 to 72 hours after their visit to gauge their satisfaction and to follow up with their condition. Another satisfaction measure is patients' intent to return to the CCC or to visit one of the operator's other sites. Information regarding how patients learned about the CCC can also be useful, as it reflects which marketing efforts have been most effective.

Provider satisfaction is also of interest to CCC management. Operators may wish to periodically assess work satisfaction to determine what staff may need to help them provide better care to patients.

THE CONVENIENT CARE CLINIC AS PART OF A LARGER NETWORK

Many CCCs are opened by chains or by larger organizations that can also include hospitals, insurance-based primary care provider offices with standard business hours, and community clinics. Operators of these larger organizations will want to know the impact of the new clinic site on overall operations, particularly, whether it is meeting the goal of bringing new customers both to the new site, and, through word of mouth, to the operators' other sites. Measures to monitor include community awareness of the operator, perhaps by tabulating client zip codes to see where the most patients are coming from. Many operators, after the new clinic has been open for a while, use focus groups or in-store interviews to better assess consumer familiarity with the new clinic, the operator's general services, and their impressions of the operator overall.

Many patients of the new clinic are likely to be customers of the operator's other service sites as well. Thus, clinics need to have in place documented processes for maintaining continuity of care across sites. EHRs, e-prescribing, and other health IT are some of the best ways to ensure that patient medical records are up-to-date at all times, no matter which location the patient is visiting.

CONCLUSION

Health care operators are under persistent pressure to meet rising patient demand despite ever-scarcer resources. In the face of tight budgets, increasing need, and the health reform mandates, many operators are realizing that they must expand their capacity to serve existing patients or to bring in new patients to medical homes, and serve patients in more cost-effective, high-quality ways. Although return on investment isn't always immediate, CCCs are proving to be a profitable way for many clinic operators to meet these new demands and achieve their goals.

17

Measuring Customer Satisfaction—Understanding the Consumer Mindset

PAUL H. KECKLEY

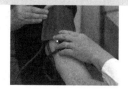

In 1969, the American Broadcasting Company (ABC) television network launched a new prime time series with its storyline centered on the professional and extracurricular dynamics of primary care medicine. Robert Young, the venerable "father" in the successful series *Father Knows Best* was tapped to play Dr. Marcus Welby in *Marcus Welby, M.D.* From 1969 to 1976, *Marcus Welby, M.D.* was a ratings hit in its time slot, largely the result of Young's portrayal of primary care as Americans imagined it—competent, compassionate, and accessible.

To older Baby Boomers and today's older adults, the depiction of Dr. Marcus Welby is still the prototype: a personable primary care physician (PCP) who appears competent and caring. But to younger populations, the prototype is changing. And with it the definition of satisfaction associated with primary care services.

CURRENT STATE OF SATISFACTION WITH PRIMARY CARE

Primary care is viewed as a physician-centered professional service in most areas of the United States, the exception being urban and rural underserved areas where nurse practitioners have been the predominant provider of primary care services. Since 2009, satisfaction with primary care has remained consistently high among U.S. adults, even as health care costs have increased and 1 million Americans lost commercial insurance coverage through their employers.[1]

The Deloitte Center for Health Solutions survey results, as seen in Table 17.1, indicate that:

- Almost four out of five U.S. adults say they have a PCP relationship
- Three of four of these U.S. adults are satisfied with the relationship
- Although satisfaction with the overall system of care in the United States. has eroded somewhat, perceptions about primary care remain largely unchanged

If we look more closely, however, we see an understandable indication that those without insurance coverage have a decidedly more negative view of primary care than others—perhaps because of access issues. What is notable is the use of or potential willingness to use convenient care clinics (CCC) as a primary care channel across all insurance classes (see Table 17.2).

Generational differences in the data, however, suggest that a person's stage in life is a critical factor in assessing primary care satisfaction: As individuals age, their inclination to be satisfied with their primary care relationship is higher, although opinions about other elements of the health care system and propensity to consider the use of a convenient care clinic do not vary in parallel (see Table 17.3).

Table 17.1 ■ Overall Assessment of Primary Care, U.S. Health System Performance

	2009	2010	2011	2012
Percent of consumers who have a PCP relationship	81	81	82	78
Percent of those who are satisfied with their PCP	72	71	73	76
Percent of consumers who rate their health status as				
Excellent/Very good	57	58	61	50
Good	31	30	30	34
Percent who take a prescription medication	57	56	57	51
Percent of consumers who grade overall system performance				
Favorably	20	24	22	34
Unfavorably	37	35	37	24

PCP, primary care physician.
Source: Deloitte Center for Health Solutions, 2012 Survey of U.S. Health Care Consumers.

Table 17.2 ■ Use of and Satisfaction With Primary Care, by Insurance Classification (2012)

	UNINSURED	MEDICAID	MEDICARE	EMPLOYER-BASED	DIRECT PURCHASE
Percent of consumers who have a PCP relationship	46	84	94	85	84
Percent of those who are satisfied with their PCP	65	73	85	75	81

	UNINSURED	MEDICAID	MEDICARE	EMPLOYER-BASED	DIRECT PURCHASE
Percent of consumers who rate their health status excellent or very good	41	33	43	59	66
Percent who take a prescription medication	28	61	80	50	18
Percent of consumers who grade overall system performance					
Favorably	21	43	48	33	39
Unfavorably	37	19	16	23	24
Percent of consumers who have used a convenient care clinic in the past year	8	8	10	7	8
Percent who are likely to use a convenient care clinic if they need care for a nonemergency health problem that is keeping them from going about their normal activities and their doctor is not able to see them right away	28	27	22	25	25

PCP, primary care physician.
Source: Deloitte Center for Health Solutions, 2012 Survey of U.S. Health Care Consumers.

Table 17.3 ■ **Opinions About Primary Care and the U.S. Health Care System, by Age (2012)**

	18–24 YEARS	25–44 YEARS	45–54 YEARS	55–64 YEARS	65 YEARS OR OLDER
Percent of consumers who have a PCP relationship	60	72	80	86	95
Percent of those who are satisfied with their PCP	65	69	76	80	88
Percent of consumers who rate their health status as excellent or very good	55	55	46	42	50
Percent who take a prescription medication	23	37	55	69	83
Percent of consumers who grade overall system performance					
Favorably	40	30	28	34	48
Unfavorably	20	26	29	27	15

(continued)

Table 17.3 ■ **Opinions About Primary Care and the U.S. Health Care System, by Age (2012)** *(continued)*

	18–24 YEARS	25–44 YEARS	45–54 YEARS	55–64 YEARS	65 YEARS OR OLDER
Percent of consumers who have used a convenient care clinic in the past year	9	8	7	8	9
Percent who are likely to use a convenient care clinic if they need care for a nonemergency health problem that is keeping them from going about their normal activities and their doctor is not able to see them right away	27	26	27	26	20

PCP, primary care physician.
Source: Deloitte Center for Health Solutions, 2012 Survey of U.S. Health Care Consumers.

In terms of the overall health care system, consumers see the role played by primary care in a positive light. In consumers' opinions, primary care services have considerable potential to lower overall costs and to achieve better health care outcomes and value for the money than the current system provides.

OPTION FOR IMPROVING PRIMARY CARE SERVICES	PERCENT WHO BELIEVE OPTION IS VIABLE
Lower overall health care spending if primary care is used early	62%
Better value for money if primary care is used early	61%
Better health outcomes if primary care is used early	56%

Source: Deloitte Center for Health Solutions, 2012 Survey of U.S. Health Care Consumers.

LOOKING AHEAD

Four factors are likely to change consumer expectations and use of primary care services in the United States, potentially resulting in changes in the nature of satisfaction with primary care services:

1. *Technology could enable transparency and decision support*: Mobile communication devices will routinely provide consumers with information about the quality, safety, accessibility, and convenience of primary care services they are about to use. When a decision about a course of treatment is made during teachable moments, consumers will be equipped to learn and act on information personalized to their unique genotypes and symptoms. Powerful tools that equip consumers to be activists in their own care will readily link PCPs and their patients.

Implication for satisfaction with primary care services: More data about performance (e.g., costs, quality, and access) is expected to be available to consumers for comparison shopping and active participation in treatment planning.

2. **Employers and Medicare incentives could drive payments through PCPs**: Incentives in primary care are likely to shift from fee-for-service to performance-based payments based on demonstrated effectiveness in population health management, efficiency, outcomes, and patient satisfaction. The expansion of Affordable Care Act (ACA) demonstrations and pilot programs (e.g., medical homes and accountable care organizations) to commercial populations are expected to drive primary care into a prominent gatekeeping role, sharing in demonstrable savings through effective care coordination and population health management. Notably, in assessing the mechanisms most impactful to cost containment, employers rank investments in primary care as among the most important in controlling costs (see Figure 17.1).

Implication for satisfaction with primary care services: Satisfaction with primary care could entail a wider array of choices for consumers and employers. Coordination of a broader set of primary care services could be necessary, and infrastructure to support risk-based contracting with employers and the government will likely be required.

3. **The primary care workforce is expected to expand as the scope of primary care services widens**: Pharmacists and nurse practitioners will become mainstream

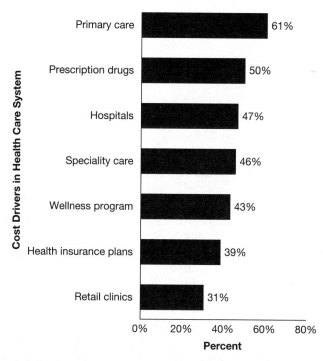

■ Provides value to health care system (rating of 8, 9, or 10)

Figure 17.1 ▨ Employers' views on health care cost drivers
Source: Deloitte Center for Health Solutions, 2012 Survey of U.S. Employers.

Table 17.4 ■ Who Do Consumers Consider to Be Their PCPs?

	2008	2012
Medical doctor	95%	87%
Nurse practitioner/physician assistant	4%	10%
Other	1%	3%

Source: Deloitte Center for Health Solutions, 2012 Survey of U.S. Health Care Consumers.

Table 17.5 ■ Select Affordable Care Act Measures of PCP Performance Satisfaction

MEASURE	DESCRIPTION
Patient satisfaction/ Patient experience with PCPs[a,b]	• Access to care (appointments and information) • Quality of physician communication • Data to show that standards of patient access and communication are being met • Patient/family satisfaction with care • Patients' rating of doctor • Access to specialists • Health promotion and education • Shared decision making • Health status/functional status
Safety/Care coordination with PCPs[c,d]	• Percent of PCPs who successfully qualify for an electronic health record incentive program payment • Use of paper or electronic charting tools to organize clinical information • Use of data to identify important diagnoses and conditions in practice • Adoption and implementation of evidence-based guidelines for three chronic or important conditions • Systematic tracking of tests and follow-up on test results • Systematic tracking of critical referrals • Performance reporting by physician or across the practice

Note: This table is not inclusive of all ACA satisfaction measures; it is specific to PCPs.
PCP, primary care physician.
Source: National Committee for Quality Assurance (NCQA), endorsed by the National Quality Forum (NQF).
[a]42 CFR Part 425.
[b]National Center for Quality Assurance (NCQA), Physician Practice Connections—Patient Centered Medical Home, www.ncqa.org/Portals/0/Programs/Recognition/Companion_Guide/Standard%208.pdf.
[c]42 CFR Part 425.
[d]NCQA Patient-Centered Medical Home (PPC-PCMH) Recognition Program, www.ncqa.org/Portals/0/PCMH%20brochure-web.pdf

providers of primary care services, and larger roles for nutritionists, psychologists, and health coaches are likely. As more consumers adopt non-allopathic forms of treatment and therapies, primary care could embrace mindfulness, counseling, medical foods, over-the-counter treatments, and a wider variety of goods and services (see Table 17.4).

Implication: Primary care is a team sport requiring a wider set of skills, core competencies, and experience. A physician-centric model will likely be inadequate.

4. *The ACA is expected to accelerate demand for primary care services:* Expanded demand for primary care services as a result of ACA insurance coverage expansion is well documented. Up to 32 million could be newly enrolled in Medicaid or health insurance exchange-based programs and will undoubtedly seek primary care services heretofore neglected.[2] Two prominent primary care programs in the ACA—medical homes and accountable care organizations—include formal metrics whereby the government will assess the performance of the care teams that serve Medicare enrollees. It is highly likely that others will be added and that safety, access, outcomes, and efficiency will be standardized so as to capture and quantify "the total patient experience." In addition, the ACA requirement that preventive health services be covered without a co-payment will likely drive consumers to more frequently use primary care services (see Table 17.5).

Implication for satisfaction with primary care services: How primary care contributes to the dual intent of the ACA to reduce costs and increase access will be closely scrutinized and evaluated by employers, consumers, and policy makers.

SATISFACTION WITH PRIMARY CARE: YESTERDAY AND TOMORROW

Given these considerations, one would expect a major shift in how the patient experience with primary care changes in coming years: Each of tomorrow's structural changes may be associated with a larger set of performance metrics standardized across regions to enable performance report cards.

OLD PARADIGM: YESTERDAY	NEW PARADIGM: TOMORROW
Central focus on an individual physician	Focus on the aggregate effectiveness of a team of primary care service providers in which the physician is a team member
Primary differentiation based on bedside manner, word of mouth, and inclusion in insurance networks negotiated by third parties	Differentiation based on quantified changes in population, costs, safety, outcomes, and user experiences
Measures of patient impressions about access and waiting times	Precise measures of competence, costs, and outcomes based on valid and reliable measures compared against local best practice benchmarks
Treatment planning driven by physician opinion	Shared decision making with consumers using clinical decision support technologies
Limited price sensitivity: costs based on co-payments and over-the-counter purchases	Increased price sensitivity: total costs absorbed by individual in context of defined contribution insurance coverage

The rise in demand for primary care services, and the scope of services providing mean satisfaction will be increasingly important. The key, however, will be what is measured and how: Tomorrow's measures are likely to be more precise on core functions and more sensitive to the unique needs of consumers, and will likely be the result more of teamwork than of an individual clinician's effort.

NOTES

1. Current Population Survey, "Health Insurance Coverage Status and Type of Coverage by State All People: 1999–2011."
2. Deloitte Center for Health Solutions, Impact of Health Care Reform on Insurance Coverage: Projection Scenarios Over 10 Years—Update 2012.

18

The Dollars and Cents of Running a Clinic

WEBSTER F. GOLINKIN AND DANIELLE BARRERA

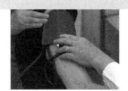

As described in earlier chapters, convenient care clinics (CCCs) have succeeded because they provide consumers with easy access to high-quality, affordable health care. As shown in Figure 18.1 research has shown that the quality of care provided at these clinics—within their limited scope of practice—is comparable with or even slightly better than the care provided at physicians' offices, urgent care clinics, and emergency rooms, and the costs are at least 40% lower (Mehrotra et al., 2009).

RAND Study Validates Benefits

Multi-year study analyzing thousands of patient visits that compared quality, cost and accessibility of convenient care clinics to that of physician offices, urgent care clinics, and ERs

Published in the September 2009 issue of the Annals of Internal Medicine, 151(5)

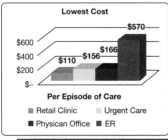

Lowest Cost

- $570
- $600
- $400
- $166
- $156
- $110
- $200
- $–

Per Episode of Care

■ Retail Clinic   Urgent Care
■ Physican Office ■ ER

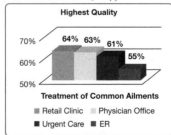

Highest Quality

- 70%
- 64% 63% 61%
- 60%
- 55%
- 50%

Treatment of Common Ailments

■ Retail Clinic   Physician Office
■ Urgent Care ■ ER

The study's primary author, Dr. Ateev Mehrota, a Professor at the University of Pittsburgh Medical School, summarized the study's findings as follows:

"Retail clinics are more convenient for patients, less costly and provide care that is of equal quality"

Figure 18.1 ■ RAND Study.

The affordability of CCCs is possible due to lower costs associated with a limited scope of practice and lower-cost staffing and marketing models. However, fixed costs are high and margins on most services offered by CCCs are thin, so high patient volume and operational efficiency are critical to achieving profitability. Thus, clinicians who staff these clinics must function as business managers and practice builders, as well as caregivers.

Although most of this chapter will be devoted to the economics of running a CCC, it is important to remember that clinic profits must ultimately recoup the initial costs of building and equipping the clinic (see Table 18.1). These costs can range from $50,000 to more than $150,000, depending on clinic size, configuration, and equipment. Although these capital expenses are lower than those for most other primary care outlets, they are still substantial, and the physical characteristics of a clinic, as well as its host store's location and the clinic's position within the store, can have a significant impact on profitability. A clinic with two or more examination rooms and a fully functional restroom located in the front of a store that is shopped by thousands of consumers daily who fit the demographic profile of CCC users may be more likely to be successful than a small clinic located in the back of a store with less foot traffic.

Table 18.1 ■ Sample CCC Profit and Loss (P&L) Statement

SAMPLE RediClinic MONTHLY CLINIC PROFIT AND LOSS STATEMENT	
Revenues	
Office visits	$75,245.70
Preventive visits	1,475.00
Immunizations	7,594.42
Laboratory revenues	2,523.38
Total revenues	$86,838.50
Product costs	
Medical supplies	$3,230.61
Vaccine cost	2,631.79
Laboratory fees	1,998.98
Gross margins	
Office visits	$72,015.09
Preventive visits	1,475.00
Immunizations	4,962.63
Laboratory revenues	524.40
Gross margin	$78,977.12

SAMPLE REDICLINIC MONTHLY CLINIC PROFIT AND LOSS STATEMENT	
Variable costs	
Clinic office supplies	$1,300.40
Bank charges	1,060.58
Bad debt/write-offs	(1,145.71)
Managed care billing expense	5,101.19
Clinic waste disposal	0.00
Total variable costs	$6,316.46
Variable margin	$73,056.66
Fixed costs	
Personnel related	$27,870.59
Medical director (oversight)	3,240.00
Contract services—cleaning	0.00
Staff CEU expense	0.00
Other training and education—COS	0.00
Clinic shipping cost	28.99
Clinic's rent	3,390.00
Clinic communications	1,494.48
Malpractice insurance	352.35
Cash short/over	0.00
Repairs and maintenance	205.68
Other/miscellaneous	0.00
Travel and entertainment	304.70
Clinic overhead	32.27
Permits, taxes, etc.	22.52
Total fixed costs	$36,941.58
Clinic profit	$36,115.08
Statistics	
Clinic operating days	29.00
Clinic operating hours	336.00

(continued)

Table 18.1 ■ Sample CCC Profit and Loss (P&L) Statement *(continued)*

SAMPLE REDICLINIC MONTHLY CLINIC PROFIT AND LOSS STATEMENT	
Patient stats	
Flu encounters	0
Office visits	1,226
Preventive visits	25
Immunizations visits	53
Laboratory visits	39
Total encounters	1,343
Gross margin per patient	
Office visits	$58.74
Preventive visits	$59.00
Immunizations	$93.63
Laboratory	$13.45
Gross margin per patient	$58.93
Variable margin per patient	$54.24
Pricing and breakeven	
Realized pricing	$64.76
Average patients per day	46.45
Patients per hour (PPH)	4.01
Cost of service metrics	
Personnel cost per patient	$20.69
Total clinic cost per patient	$37.95
Labor as ratio of revenues	0.32
Bad debt as ratio of revenues	−0.01
Labor details	
Biweekly wages	$20,618.04
Payroll accrual	(463.97)
Payroll tax	$1,162.25
Bonus	$2,074.83

SAMPLE RediClinic MONTHLY CLINIC PROFIT AND LOSS STATEMENT	
Holiday pay	$0.00
Paid time off	$1,594.54
Benefits	$3,573.32
Overtime	(688.42)
On-call payroll	0.00
Other payroll related	0.00
Total	$27,870.59

One of the main reasons that CCCs have been successful is that they are convenient. Part of their convenience comes from being located in a drugstore, grocery store, or big box outlet where consumers shop on a regular basis. Another aspect of their convenience is that appointments are generally not necessary, visits take about 15 minutes (due to the limited scope of practice), and patients can get their prescriptions filled in the in-store pharmacy. An additional convenience of the clinics is that they are generally open 7 days a week, with extended weekday hours. Although this accessibility has been very important to the success of CCCs, it is challenging from a business standpoint because it means that the clinics may need to be staffed for up to 75 hours per week, or more, whether or not there is a high volume of patients. Because labor is by far the largest cost of running a clinic, this means that clinics have high fixed costs, which also include the costs of physician oversight, rent, and other items that are part of individual clinic or corporate cost structures.

It usually takes 15 to 25 patients per day to cover a CCC's high fixed costs, as well as variable costs for medical supplies, vaccines, lab testing, billing expenses, bad debt, marketing, and other items. Incremental patient volume over a clinic's breakeven point is highly profitable, but exceeding the breakeven point 7 days a week, 52 weeks a year is not easy, particularly during the first few years of a clinic's operations. The most cost-effective way for a new clinic to generate patient volume is to leverage its host store's existing shoppers, primarily through in-store and external signage. Efforts also should be made to ensure that consumers and employers in a store's trade area are aware of the clinic, its services, and benefits. Media advertising can be effective as well, but usually not until a clinic operator has a large number of clinics and geographic coverage in a market.

The CCC value proposition of quality, convenience, and affordability is generally sufficient to get consumers to try the clinics, but the most important driver of patient volume is ultimately patient satisfaction. Patients who are satisfied with their experience will return for other services and will tell their family members and friends. Conversely, dissatisfied patients will share their negative impressions, sometimes even more vocally than "raving fans." There are many drivers of patient satisfaction, including the quality of care, staff friendliness and professionalism, patient wait time, clinic cleanliness, and accurate billing and collections process. These are the things that generally make or break a CCC, which is as much of a retail business as it is a health care delivery outlet.

Although wait time and cycle time are important drivers of patient satisfaction, they are also critical drivers of profitability. Particularly during periods of the year when seasonal demand for CCCs is naturally strong—such as back-to-school in August through September and cough/cold/flu season in October through March—it is important to treat patients quickly without compromising the quality of care, because long wait times are inconsistent with the convenient care value proposition. There are many keys to maximizing patient throughput, but one of the most important is to leverage health IT. Electronic medical records (EMRs) that include both clinical and billing components can significantly reduce the amount of staff time devoted to administrative tasks. Online preregistration and electronic self-registration kiosks are also used to reduce cycle time and maximize the amount of time that is devoted to patient care.

Another driver of patient volume is a clinic's scope of services. Most clinics treat common medical conditions such as conjunctivitis, otitis media, pharyngitis, sinusitis, and urinary tract infections, and many provide preventive services, including screenings and medical tests, immunizations, and basic physical examinations. Preventive services are particularly important to profitability because demand for them is growing and is year-round, which helps to attract patients during the off-season months of April to July when incidence of acute-episodic conditions wanes. Some operators, including RediClinic, augment their preventive service offerings with disease and lifestyle management programs such as weight management and smoking cessation. If properly designed, these programs can be delivered by the same nurse practitioners and physician assistants who provide a clinic's core services in the same 15- to 20-minute visit time frames that are standard for other services.

In addition to patient volume, another key driver of profitability is the average size of each patient transaction, or average ticket. For cash-paying patients and services not usually covered by insurance, the average ticket at most CCCs can be high enough to achieve acceptable margins on each patient visit while still being significantly lower than other health care delivery outlets. However, today and increasingly in the future, most CCC patients and services will be covered by insurance. This means the average ticket is and will be largely determined by rates negotiated with third-party payers, including both commercial and government payers. Generally speaking, CCCs will have difficulty achieving sustained profitability if their average ticket is less than $65.00.

The importance of third-party payers to the success of a CCC poses two challenges to clinic operators and staff members. First, while third-party payers have increasingly embraced CCCs because of their high-quality care, high levels of patient/member satisfaction, and lower costs, negotiating mutually beneficial agreements with these large organizations requires clinic operators to make a strong business case for the value they are providing. Second, it is critical that any staff responsible for registering patients have a system for determining at the point of service whether a patient is covered by a contracted plan, whether the plan covers the service being rendered, whether the patient has met his or her deductible, and thus how much of a co-payment or other amount to collect from the patient. Collecting the right amount from each

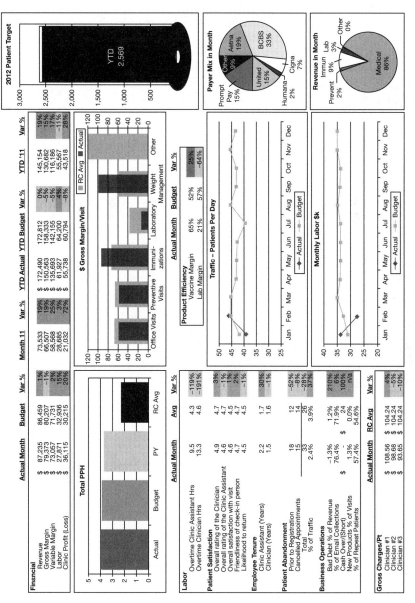

Figure 18.2 ▮ Sample monthly clinic dashboard.

patient at the point of service is one of the most challenging aspects of running a CCC, as there are many variables and usually not much time for the person registering a patient to make the correct decision.

As you can see, although the CCC value proposition is simple, delivering it in a profitable manner is not easy. It is not unusual for a clinic operator to spend $300,000 or more to open a clinic and fund operating losses to cash flow breakeven, and it can take up to 2 years or more for profitability to be achieved. It takes a dedicated and experienced team of people at the corporate and clinic levels to achieve this milestone, but providing consumers with easy access to high-quality, affordable health care can be as rewarding financially as it is in many other ways.

19

Research and Quality, Cost, and Access

CAROLINE G. RIDGWAY

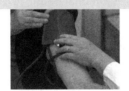

Convenient care is a relatively new industry, still developing measurable outcomes; as such, the body of third-party literature around retail-based convenient care has been somewhat slow to accumulate. However, a number of studies have been published in recent years, which tend to validate the purported value proposition of the model: affordable, accessible, and high quality. Initial concerns around poor quality of care and the potential for conflict of interest and disruption to continuity of care have largely been disproven. However, the long-term contributions of this care model are yet to be fully known. For example, a more recent concern is that the clinics, because of the very accessibility and affordability that define them, will induce overutilization among patients, thereby increasing, rather than reducing, costs to the system. There have been no reports indicating that this is definitively the case, but the fact remains that convenient care is still a relatively new entrant to the health care marketplace and more time is needed to ascertain its true role and impact.

AFFORDABILITY

A central founding principle behind convenient care is the notion of cost-effectiveness and affordability. As is discussed elsewhere in this textbook in greater detail, the first convenient care clinics (CCCs) were founded as cash only. The relatively no-frills business model (e.g., limited scope of services, one provider with no administrative staff, and small physical footprint) contributed to low prices, which operators backed up by offering full transparency of costs. Gradually, clinic operators began contracting with insurance companies, to the extent that today, the majority of payers include CCCs within their networks.

Although the baseline cost of care at CCCs appears lower than other care settings, there has long been concern, as alluded to in the introductory paragraph, that the enhanced user-friendliness of these clinics will induce overutilization among consumers who previously would not have sought care at all or who would have delayed care to be seen by their primary care provider, thus effectively driving up overall system costs. In addition, there has been speculation that patients of CCCs would seek subsequent care more often than patients of primary care physician practices, also increasing utilization costs. To date, however, research has supported the claim that retail-based clinics are substantially lower in cost than other traditional points of care, including primary care physician practices, urgent care centers, and emergency departments, and that patients are not using this or other points of care significantly more frequently as a consequence of the increased access.

The first major third-party study to be published about the question of cost of care in retail settings (Thygeson, Van Vorst, Maciosek, & Solberg, 2008) reported on claims data for five diagnoses (pink eye, ear infection, tonsillitis/pharyngitis, sinusitis, and urinary tract infection [UTI]) from a Minnesota insurer. On the question of average total cost per episode, the authors concluded that the CCC was $51 less expensive than an urgent care clinic, $55 less than a visit to a physician office, and $279 less than the cost of going to an emergency room for treatment of conditions in question. The authors reported a slight increase in the number of CCC patients who sought additional care after their visit (2%) but noted that (1) they could not definitively determine the cause of this increase (such as appropriate referrals of patients for care outside of the CCC scope) and (2) increases in cost during the study period were primarily a function of increased costs overall and not an increase in the volume of patient visits.

A subsequent study (Mehrotra et al., 2009) examined claims data from the same insurer and confirmed the initial finding of lower per-episode costs. The study authors sought to evaluate the costs of an entire episode of care, which they defined as having concluded when no further services were billed for 30 days, for ear infections, pharyngitis, and UTI, as compared with physician office visits, urgent care centers, and emergency rooms. Episodes of care included evaluation and management visits, pharmaceutical costs, laboratory and imaging, inpatient care, and other costs. Across each diagnosis, CCC costs were significantly lower than were costs for the other sites considered; the average cost at a retail-based clinic was $110 for the entire episode of care, $166 at physician offices, $156 at urgent care centers, and $570 at an emergency room. Thygeson and colleagues found a slight bump in repeat visits for users of CCCs; these authors did not observe meaningful differences in the rate of follow-up visits among CCCs, physician practices, and urgent care centers.

Other reports and trends have supported the apparent cost-effectiveness of convenient care. Notably, in 2008, BlueCross BlueShield of Minnesota elected to eliminate co-pays for many of their enrollees who visited CCCs, citing consumer use of the clinics and cost savings of $1.2 million in 2007 (Wyant, 2008). In a May 2012 report, PricewaterhouseCoopers surmised that retail-based clinics and other alternatives to traditional primary care are contributing to decreasing costs, as consumers look to options with greater affordability, convenience, and transparency (Health Research Institute, 2012). Increasing deductibles and co-pays may ultimately prove the final counterbalance to the concern that a low-cost care alternative stimulates overutilization of resources; as costs of care are further shifted onto the consumer and if providers are to be held accountable for the care they provide, options such as CCCs will only become more attractive in the future.

ACCESSIBILITY

Convenience appears to be a primary driver of the use of retail-based clinics. A recent study determined that overall use of CCCs has increased fourfold from 2007 to 2009, with the number of annual patient visits increasing from 1.48 million in 2007 to 3.52 million in 2008 and 5.97 million in 2009 (Mehrotra & Lave, 2012). Analyses showed that 44.4% of CCC visits were on weekends and during weekday hours when physician offices were typically closed, indicating that many patients preferentially utilize retail-based care services when it is convenient for them, rather than waiting to see a primary care provider during standard office hours. The accessibility of the clinics may also be contributing to better uptake of preventive services such as influenza vaccinations. These authors estimate that 2.4 million people, accounting for not quite 2% of all of those who received an influenza vaccine during the 2009 to 2010 flu season, received that service at a CCC.

Other research has demonstrated the value that users of CCCs appear to place on convenience and accessibility. A 2009 study examining proximity of the U.S. population to existing CCCs as of August 2008 ($n = 982$) estimated that nearly 30% (28.7) lived within a 10-minute drive of a clinic location (Rudavsky, Pollack, & Mehrotra, 2009). For residents of urban areas, that proportion grew to 35.8%. A 2011 report analyzing claims data concluded that convenience was a significant predictor of CCC use, with consumers who lived within 1 mile of a clinic location being 7.5% more likely to use its services than did people who lived 10 to 20 miles away (Ashwood et al., 2011). Another study, using direct patient interview to assess reasons for clinic visits, confirmed that nearness of the clinic and minimal wait time were both highly rated by patients as reasons for their decision about where to seek care (Wang, Ryan, McGlynn, & Mehrotra, 2010).

Early prognostications by industry founders that CCCs would be a boon for underserved communities because of their low cost and convenience have not so far been supported in the literature. The only study to specifically address this question found an underrepresentation of CCCs in census tracts identified as medically underserved (Pollack & Armstrong, 2009). Demographic research has suggested a higher likelihood of clinic use among those with higher median household incomes (Ashwood et al., 2011). However, nearly 30% of clinic users pay in cash and nearly 65% report not having a usual source of care (Mehrotra & Lave, 2012). Consequently, it appears that the clinics are attracting patients of all demographics regardless of their geographic proximity.

QUALITY CARE

Questions about the quality of care provided at CCCs have been posed since the earliest days of the industry. As soon as the model began to proliferate, physician organizations in particular began to raise concerns about the potential for subpar care to be delivered in the clinics and pushed for regulation of the industry to ensure that particular standards would be upheld. Although quality of care can be difficult to quantify, a variety of research studies have been published that support the contention that CCCs are meeting high standards of care.

One of the earliest publications on the topic of convenient care issued a strong rebuke to the contention that the clinics were delivering poor quality care (Woodburn, Smith, & Nelson, 2007). Looking specifically at adherence to clinical guidelines for the treatment of acute pharyngitis across all patient ages, the authors observed a rate of 99.05% adherence for the 39,530 patients with a negative rapid strep test and 99.75% adherence for the 13,471 patients with a positive rapid strep test. A small number of patients (n = 414) were prescribed antibiotics despite not falling within the guidelines; practitioners documented their reasoning for such prescribing 44.89% of the time. Of the patients whose rapid strep tests were negative, 38,810 had additional laboratory testing; 3,395 of those came back positive, 96.2% of which resulted in antibiotic prescribing. The authors were able to conclude that the use of practice guidelines in conjunction with electronic health records (EHRs), supplemented with adequate provider training, did contribute to enhanced quality of care.

A later study also tracked high rates of adherence among CCC practitioners (Jacoby, Crawford, Chaudhari, & Goldfarb, 2010). The authors used EHR data to examine appropriateness of care of pediatric patients in CCCs for pharyngitis and upper respiratory infection, based on adherence to HEDIS (Healthcare Effectiveness Data and Information Set) metrics. Overall findings were that practitioners appropriately followed recommended practices 88.35% of the time for URI and 92.72% of the time for pharyngitis. Primary reasons for writing an antibiotic for URI without clinical indication were parental request and clinical judgment about the patient's clinical presentation. Documentation error in the electronic medical record contributed to approximately one quarter (24%) of failure to adhere in the treatment of pharyngitis; the authors speculate that this was a main contributor to the lower overall adherence rating for pharyngitis as compared with URI.

Mehrotra and colleagues, in the same 2009 study in which they determined that CCCs rated lower on a cost-per-episode basis than did traditional providers, also observed that the quality of the care provided in the clinics was similar to that in physician offices and urgent care centers and better than the care provided by emergency departments. Quality was measured based on a variety of metrics, including the RAND Corporation's Quality Assurance Tools and guidelines from the American Academy of Pediatrics, American Academy of Family Physicians, and Infectious Diseases Society of America. Notably, as it relates to earlier suspicions by detractors of convenient care that the clinics would drive increased antibiotic prescribing, the authors found no disparity in the rate of prescribing across the study group. Similarly, preventive care was offered at similar rates by CCCs, primary physician practices, and urgent care centers indicating that patients are not missing crucial opportunities for preventive intervention based on their decision to visit a retail-based clinic for care.

CONCLUSION

This chapter reflects a brief review of the primary literature published to date about the retail-based CCI. Although there is ample consistency among the conclusions drawn by the authors of the various studies as to the apparent benefits of this model of care, as mentioned at the outset of the chapter, the convenient care industry is still in its nascence as it compares with established modes of health care delivery, and its long-term role in health care is yet to be fully defined.

For instance, recent research considers that CCCs may be having a negative impact on continuity of care, a concern long posed by physician organizations and detractors of convenient care, by discouraging future use of primary care providers among CCC users (Reid et al., 2012). The study authors compared subsequent use of either CCCs or primary care practices depending on whether the patient initiated care with a CCC or primary care practice. Use of CCCs was found to be associated with less future contact with primary care practices, although no difference was found in rates of preventive care.

The meaning of these findings, however, is open to interpretation. Although it is likely that proponents of traditional, office-based, physician-based care models would look at this as evidence that CCCs are directly contributing to the erosion of the quality of primary care in the United States, an alternative explanation is that the way many Americans access and consume health care is fundamentally changing, and that if primary care practices could equal CCCs in terms of their efficiency, timeliness of care, and cost effectiveness, more patients would seek care there. It also remains the case that a large percentage of CCC patients report not having a primary care relationship, in which case the notion of continuity is moot. Furthermore, the study authors note that while their results indicate a decrease in continuity as defined by the frequency of visits to a care setting, they cannot determine the extent to which continuity may be preserved by the appropriate sharing of patient records, underscoring the importance of communication among providers and the use of electronic records systems.

Despite the uncertainty, what can be comfortably concluded is that the industry has drawn the attention of influential stakeholders within health care nationally and has spurred needed dialog about alternatives to care that establish that affordability, accessibility, and quality are not mutually exclusive traits.

20

Quality Metrics and Initiatives in the Clinic Setting

JANICE M. MILLER AND DAVID B. NASH

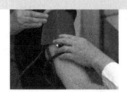

Everyone at some point is a consumer, and all consumers want to know that they are getting sufficient quality and value from the goods or services they pay for. We want to know that the products we purchase meet industry standards. For example, we expect that the dashboard of a new car will include a speedometer and a fuel gauge that are relaying accurate information to guide our driving behaviors and choices. In health care, the stakes for the consumer are higher and the margin for error is low. For clinicians providing care, the consumers are patients, their families, and insurers. Consumers deserve to know that the health care they receive and pay for is a good value and meets high-quality standards. Health care quality is defined as "the degree to which health services for individuals and populations increase the likelihood of desired health outcomes and are consistent with current professional knowledge" (Institute of Medicine, 2000). The purpose of this chapter is to describe quality measurement, the quality infrastructure of convenient care clinics, and the importance of quality to the industry.

MEASURING QUALITY

One way to evaluate the quality of health care is by using measures or "quality metrics." A quality measure or metric is a tool to measure what tests and services are provided to patients with specific illnesses. It allows for quality of care provided to be quantified and compared against an evidence-based standard or expectation (Agency for Healthcare Research and Quality [AHRQ], 2012). AHRQ has compiled a database of quality measures, the National Quality Measures Clearinghouse (NQMC), that identifies the following three general purposes of quality measurement: to improve quality, to produce accountability for care, and to use in research. Most quality metrics evaluate structure, processes, or outcomes, such as the performance of recommended testing or outcomes of care such as patient satisfaction or control of blood pressure. Quality metrics identify problems and opportunities for continuous improvement. Reevaluation is then possible by comparing the most recent set of measurements with the baseline. The most efficient way to evaluate care quality is to compare the care provided against a benchmark or standard of care.

Quality metrics differ by setting. Hospital quality metrics include measures such as administration of an antibiotic before surgery. Measures in the outpatient setting include measures for patients with diabetes such as timely performance of annual tests. Similarly, measures exist for the acute illnesses often seen in convenient care clinics, such as administering a rapid strep test or taking a throat culture when a streptococcal infection is suspected. There are also measures of screening and preventive care such as immunizations and cancer screenings. Similarly, there are mechanisms to ensure quality by evaluating whether services were appropriately withheld, such as withholding antibiotics for viral upper respiratory infections. Customarily, quality measures are reported for groups of patients as the percentage of patients who received appropriate care. In general, the higher the calculated percentage, the better the quality of care.

WHO SETS THE STANDARDS FOR QUALITY?

Returning to the car analogy, there are certain standards that we take for granted. For example, the gas pedal is always to the right of the brake pedal, a standard set by the automotive industry. Health care standards are set by various expert panels and professional organizations, such as the American Academy of Pediatrics (AAP), the United States Preventive Services Task Force (USPSTF), and the National Quality Forum (NQF). Standards are based on guidelines developed from evidence that demonstrates what components should be included in patients' care. Standards of care for defined illnesses include guidelines for assessing, diagnosing, and treating patients to ensure appropriate care and management. They often include algorithms that help clinicians make decisions at the point of care. One key to improving quality is minimizing variation in how care is provided. A second key is defining expectations for quality of care when care processes are being developed. Here the goal is to encourage the provider to follow a standard of care just as reflexively as we reach for the gas pedal on the right of the car floor.

HEDIS

On a national scale, the Healthcare Effectiveness and Data Information Set (HEDIS) is a widely accepted 76-measure reporting mechanism used for health plans to report quality measures; pneumococcal vaccination rates are one example of a HEDIS measure that is relevant to convenient care clinics (CCCs). HEDIS measures provide a reference point or benchmark against which practices can compare their quality reports. They are updated annually by the National Committee for Quality Assurance (NCQA) in its *State of Health Care Quality* report (NCQA, 2012).

CERTIFICATION AND ACCREDITATION

To identify whether health care entities and their providers conform to standards, certain organizations with subject matter expertise have been established to confer approval. The organizations are then certified or accredited in their respective fields.

There is a long history of certification and accreditation of health care quality. In 1951, the Joint Commission on Accreditation of Hospitals (JCAHO; now The Joint Commission) was initiated to reform hospitals based on the outcomes of care. The Joint Commission evaluated a hospital's ability to care for patients safely and effectively, but has since evolved and expanded to areas outside the hospital setting. In 1985, the Accreditation Commission for Health Care (ACHC) was established to provide accreditation for small home care and hospice agencies (ACHC, 2012). Numerous other entities exist with dual best-practice education and accreditation roles, such as the Utilization Review Accreditation Commission and the NCQA for both hospital and ambulatory settings.

CONVENIENT CARE ASSOCIATION

Most retail-based clinics are members of the Convenient Care Association (CCA). The CCA is the professional organization of the various companies and health systems that provide care in a retail setting. The CCA has had a commitment to quality and safety since its inception in 2006. To foster a culture of quality, and to promote common standards throughout the retail industry, member clinics must meet CCA Quality and Safety Standards including developing and using operational policies and procedures.

In an effort to maintain objectivity and oversight, the CCA requires a third-party certification or accreditation of the clinics' implementation of CCA standards and recommendation for or against the clinic's membership in the organization. The Joint Commission also identifies elements, based on their Comprehensive Accreditation Manual for Ambulatory Care (CAMAC), of CCC performance that must be met for accreditation and makes these elements available to CCC operators.

Shortly after the inception of the CCA, the Jefferson School of Population Health (JSPH) was selected as the third-party entity to develop and conduct reviews to ascertain the degree of conformity of member clinics to the CCA Quality and Safety Standards (Hansen-Turton, Ridgway, Ryan, & Nash, 2009). The initial application process requires documentation of policies and procedures consistent with CCA standards and documentation of performance of the following:

- Credentialing of providers
- Ongoing quality monitoring
- Coordination of care with outside providers (copy of visit notes faxed to primary care provider if the patient requests)
- Provision to the patient of a written visit record with clear discharge instructions
- Encouragement of patients to form relationships and follow up with primary care physicians (PCPs), and making referrals as indicated
- Health promotion and preventive screening information
- Compliance with regulatory standards (such as HIPAA, OSHA, and CDC guidelines)
- Use of electronic health records (EHRs)
- Peer and collaborating physician chart review
- Maintenance of a safe, infection-free environment
- Mechanisms to empower patients to make informed choices
- Emergency response procedures

Once the documentation is received and reviewed by JSPH, and found to conform to CCA quality standards, a recommendation is made for the CCC's certification. Certification is valid for 2 years.

RECERTIFICATION

Recertification is achieved through a variety of formats and often with the same entity through which initial certification was achieved. The predominant goal is to identify opportunities to develop and enhance quality improvement strategies. Quality initiatives undertaken since initial certification are submitted as evidence, as are minutes from quality improvement committee meetings and quality reports generated by the clinic. Examples include waiting time reports, patient satisfaction surveys, and evidence of appropriateness of care based on chart review. Action plans to address areas of deficiencies must also be submitted. Furthermore, as all clinics are required to utilize EHRs, they must demonstrate how the EHR is used in a meaningful way (referred to as "meaningful use" in the 2009 American Recovery and Reinvestment Act), such as how the EHR interfaces with other providers, how the EHR provides warnings such as potential drug interactions, or how the EHR is utilized to track quality data.

EVIDENCE OF QUALITY OF CARE IN A CONVENIENT CARE CLINIC

Numerous studies have documented the high quality of care provided in CCCs. Mehrotra et al. (2009) compared the cost and quality of care provided for otitis media, urinary tract infections, pharyngitis, and preventive care treated in a

CCC. The authors compared CCC data to that of physician offices, urgent care centers, and emergency rooms: Overall costs were significantly lower in CCCs. Aggregate data on quality metrics were best for CCCs, though not statistically different from those for physician offices or urgent care centers. Comparison with emergency departments demonstrated statistically superior quality in CCCs for the aforementioned conditions. Woodburn et al. (2007) found that nurse practitioners (NPs) and physician assistants (PAs) in the retail setting adhered to guidelines more than 99% of the time for testing and treatment for pharyngitis. Jacoby et al. (2010) studied data from visits to one member of the CCA, Take Care Health Systems (TCHS), over a 2-year period. Appropriate treatment was accomplished for children with upper respiratory infections in 88% of visits and for pharyngitis in 93% of visits. Both results surpassed HEDIS benchmarks.

How Does Quality Happen?

When tragedies occur such as a jetliner crash or the collapse of large financial institutions, we invariably ask: "How did this happen?" Given the evidence for superb quality achievement in the CCC, we must ask the same question. Identifying the components of success at the granular and structural levels permits reproducibility of the components as well as recognizing areas for ongoing improvement.

To demonstrate how one convenient care clinic proactively incorporated quality measurement, let us look at one CCA member, TCHS. In many nonretail health care settings, the EHR is retrofitted into the existing practice structure. The CCC industry, however, gained momentum at the same time that the value of EHRs was becoming recognized. As a result, TCHS, with its long commitment to quality and safety, designed a patient-centric EHR that incorporated quality measurement at the forefront. From TCHS's inception, each exam room was equipped with a computer that houses evidence-based standards, guidelines, and the EHRs. Detailed information is recorded as providers use the EHR during the visit.

Quality Metrics at TCHS

Each provider entry contributes to the database of diagnosis codes, tests conducted during the visit, and therapies prescribed. TCHS can rapidly determine a provider's history, including the number of patients he or she treated for a particular diagnosis and the frequency with which recommended activities were performed and therapies prescribed. Regional NP managers review the data frequently to identify deviance from standards. In addition to evaluating provider-based data, reviews can be conducted for specific quality metrics, such as how frequently urine cultures are procured for patients with urinary tract infections. In this manner, aggregate quality trends for the entire system, the region, specific clinics, and providers can be determined and improved if indicated. Regional NP managers who oversee the quality data provide performance reports to the providers quarterly, at in-person group meetings where goals and improvement strategies are disseminated.

Evidence-Based Guidelines

Each examination room computer permits access to detailed evidence-based guidelines for conditions treated in the CCC. Algorithms serve as clinical decision aids at points of care, yet providers may choose to individualize therapy as indicated. Diagnostic tests are suggested, as are recommended therapies, doses, and lengths of treatment, and follow-up suggestions are available. Providers can also use the EHR without referring to the protocols. The system enables queries such as the safety of vaccines in pregnancy. The EHR also provides recommendations and contraindications for vaccinations, which constitute a large percentage of CCC visits (Mehrotra & Lave, 2012). Guidelines are based on standards from nationally recognized organizations and approved by content experts.

Training and Orientation

Providers new to the TCHS undergo 6 to 8 weeks of training and orientation with a preceptor. During this time, they gain familiarity with guidelines of care and with the EHR. CCA standards and how they are specifically implemented at TCHS are reinforced. A variety of ongoing learning activities are available to providers through the examination room terminals. Many of the TCHS learning modules offer continuing education credits that may be applied to licensure requirements.

Peer Review

Oversight in any organization improves accuracy, transparency, and accountability. Historically, lack of oversight and standards has been blamed for financial and moral collapses. Oversight in health care increases the likelihood that providers meet established standards. Each provider in the TCHS conducts reviews of their peers' visit records. Ten percent of each provider's charts are evaluated by peers in different geographic locations of the country. This "peer review" permits providers to grade each other's performance as reflected in various sections of the visit and examination note. For example, reviewers are asked whether the relevant medical and social histories are thorough and whether the diagnosis and treatment are correct. A provider has the opportunity to rebut the review if extenuating or special circumstances indicated a deviation in care. Ongoing quarterly reports are generated for all providers. The rare provider not meeting HEDIS standards is reeducated for performance improvement.

COLLABORATING PHYSICIAN REVIEW

The degree of NP and PA practice autonomy varies by state. In states requiring collaborative agreements, a portion of the providers' charts are reviewed by collaborating physicians. Criteria for evaluation are similar to those described earlier in the discussion of peer review. Collaborating physicians have the opportunity to comment on and grade the care that is documented. Similarly, results are returned to individual providers and are available in summary form to regional managers.

SUMMARY

Certification and accreditation processes are integral to the successful achievement of CCA's goals. CCA's longstanding and ongoing commitment to quality and safety is demonstrated through a variety of means, and its Quality and Safety Standards set expectations. Clinic investment in developing a culture of quality and safety is evident through training and orientation programs, EHRs, peer reviews, certification processes, and quality reporting mechanisms. This constellation of activities in convenient care clinics serves as a model for improving quality of care.

ACKNOWLEDGMENTS

Thanks to Bettina Berman, RN, BSN, CPHQ, Albert Crawford, PhD, Richard Jacoby, MD, and Valerie Pracilio, MPH for their review of the chapter and suggestions; to Janice Clarke, RN, for demonstration of the CCA certification process and documentation; and to Patricia Jacobs, MSN, FNP-C for demonstration of Take Care Clinic quality initiatives and reporting activities.

21

Collaboration and Partnership in the Convenient Care Setting

WILLIAM D. WRIGHT AND EILEEN STELLEFSON MYERS

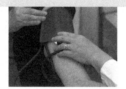

The role of physician collaboration within convenient care clinics has evolved over time. Because convenient care clinics (CCCs) are generally led by nurse practitioners (NPs) and physician assistants (PAs), many of the clinical activities (diagnosing, treating, and prescribing) are only possible with the participation of licensed physicians who are also referred to as medical directors; the level and degree of physician interaction in the daily operations of a clinic are functions of regulatory considerations and of the clinic operator's operating model. Some jurisdictions require extensive direct (on-site) supervision of NPs and PAs, whereas other states grant near-independent practice.

As new models of care delivery are developed (accountable care organizations, patient-centered medical homes), CCCs serve as a critical entry point into the care continuum. Because of the need for coordination and vertical integration, clinics and large practice groups and institutions are working in new and innovative models to promote the health and wellness of local communities. This chapter provides an overview of the basic framework and considerations of physician participation in the clinic environment and how CCCs can play an integral part in care delivery in collaboration with large practice groups and institutions.

SCOPE OF PRACTICE AND DERIVED MEDICAL AUTHORITY

Although NPs and PAs receive extensive training and advanced education, many states require such clinicians to establish a relationship with a licensed physician prior to engaging in advanced clinical treatment. State regulations define the outer parameters of the services the clinician may legally perform. The advanced clinical services (diagnosing, treatment, and prescribing) typically reside within the definition of the practice of medicine, and without a statutory exception, the practice of medicine may only be engaged by a licensed physician. In order to acknowledge the education and training of NPs and PAs, these professions are permitted an extended scope of practice, but only when accompanied by certain oversight, supervision, or collaboration with a physician.

NP—Nurse Practice Act

All nurses, whether licensed practical nurses (LPNs), registered nurses (RNs), or NPs, have inherent limits on permissible procedures. The permissible scope of nursing practice is delineated in each state's nurse practice act, the statutory documents that govern nursing professionals.[1] Although nursing professionals are accustomed to performing a wide range of clinical activities in the physicians' office or institutional setting, most clinical services performed in a CCC are beyond the natural nursing scope of practice. This presents a legal and logistical challenge to CCC operators.

In order to expand the scope of practice for NPs into a limited practice of medicine, statutes and regulations have evolved to delegate limited authority from physicians to NPs. The rules are usually developed and enforced by the state board of nursing, the board of medicine, or some combined oversight board specifically developed for advanced practice nurses. The following items are typically addressed in the delegation:

Prescriptive authority: This area is essential to a successful CCC. Some states require an NP to complete additional educational requirements or preceptorships/internships with physicians to develop safe prescribing practices. In addition, many states require NPs and physicians to enter into written agreements to document the safe prescribing practices and limits of drugs that may be prescribed (for instance, controlled substances may be more restricted than antibiotics). Some states delineate a prescription formulary that the NP must follow.

Supervision, oversight, and collaboration: States impose a variety of mechanisms to ensure meaningful interaction between physicians and NPs. The requirements vary widely from state to state and include the following:
- Mandatory on-site supervision for a percentage of open clinic hours (Texas currently requires a physician to be on site for 10% of operating hours per week)
- Mandatory chart review, either as a percentage of NP encounters per month or in certain predefined clinical circumstances (upon patient request, whenever controlled substances are prescribed)

- Periodic face-to-face meetings to review and discuss patient care and medical standards

Written protocols: Protocols articulate the obligations and responsibilities of the physician and NP. Topics often required in protocols include the following:

- Availability of physician to consult with NP (either in person or by telephone)
- Transfer of patients when acuity exceeds NP scope or in emergencies
- Coverage during times of physician unavailability
- Development of quality standards that will be used to measure clinical care
- The underlying reference materials to be used in the development of evidence-based practice

PAs

Unlike NPs, PAs are typically regulated and governed by the state boards of medicine. In some states, this alignment with medicine provides greater autonomy in clinical practice, whereas others impose additional restrictions and requirements for physician interaction. For example, Arizona regulations require periodic face-to-face conferences between physician and PA, while Arizona NPs do not have the same requirement. Other states, like Tennessee, have nearly identical rules and regulations for NP and PA practice.[2] It is critically important to consider the impact and expense of the various supervision and collaboration requirements prior to developing a business model.

FRAUD AND ABUSE CONSIDERATIONS

Because of the prohibition of payments and referrals between and among clinics and physicians, any relationship must satisfy an exception to the federal Ethics in Patient Referrals Act (commonly known as the Stark Law) and the Anti-Kickback Statute (AKS). The Stark Law prohibits a physician from having a financial relationship with another entity and referring patients to that entity for certain designated health services. Any claim submitted to the Centers for Medicare & Medicaid Services (CMS) based on a tainted referral is deemed to be a false claim, leading to liability under the False Claims Act. There are a number of exceptions that allow a physician and an entity to enter into an arms-length relationship and receive payment for services.

Both Stark and the AKS provide exceptions and safe harbor based on personal service arrangements. In order for a payment from a clinic to a physician to not be deemed impermissible, each of these must be taken into account when developing a clinic model:

1. The agreement must be in writing and signed by the parties
2. The agreement must be for at least 1 year and specify the services covered
3. The services must meet (not exceed) a legitimate business purpose
4. Payments must be fair market value and not vary based on the volume or value of Medicare or Medicaid patient referrals between the parties
5. None of the intents to pay for services can be compensable by federal health care programs
6. The services must not involve the counseling or promotion of an illegal activity under state or federal law

PARTNERING WITH THE PRIMARY CARE PHYSICIAN AND THE MEDICAL HOME

The future of health care is focused on an affordable, patient-centered system with easy access to coordinated care for the ultimate purpose of better care quality at lower cost. Care coordination has been designated as one of the six health care improvement priorities for national action by the Institute of Medicine and National Quality Forum. In the early days of retail-based care, clinics were criticized for disrupting care coordination between the clinics and patients' medical homes; however, over the past several years, relationships have been evolving between the retail health clinic and the primary care home for improved care coordination and patient care.

Establishing Relationships With Primary Care Providers

The easiest type of relationship to establish with a primary care provider (PCP) is when a patient presents at the clinic with symptoms or an illness outside the clinic's scope of services. In a triage function, a phone call to the patient's PCP provides the clinician with guidance on where to send the patient. This phone call to the PCP can prevent an unnecessary ER visit and this extra step goes a long way in establishing a positive relationship with the PCP, who may then think of the clinic when he or she needs to refer a walk-in patient who cannot be seen that day.

Many CCC patients report that they do not have a PCP; they seek care for episodic illnesses or preventive care (vaccinations, flu shots) but have no medical home. Many of these patients may not have PCPs because they lack health insurance, and CCCs can assist by providing lists of walk-in community clinics and county clinics in the area. This again helps foster relationships between local clinics and CCCs in which each recommends the other's services depending on the needs of the patient.

Even patients who do have PCPs may choose to visit CCCs for some of their care, to avoid long wait times for appointments or for urgent issues that arise outside of standard medical office hours. For some of these patients, the CCC visit may have been just for an episodic illness but may reveal unknown underlying conditions that require follow-up. Having caught the ailment early, the CCC provider can connect with the patient's PCP, forward the visit summary, and get the patient an earlier appointment and earlier treatment than she might have gotten had she just waited to see her regular provider.

Primary Care Needs CCCs

The new era of health care will ask primary care to take on the burden of treating and coordinating care for the vast majority of our population. Yet, we face a primary care shortage, both now and in the foreseeable future. In light of the shortage and increased demand, CCCs can participate in the solution in a variety of both informal and formal ways by partnering with PCPs as an integral part of the medical neighborhood.

Effective marketing of a new CCC should include reaching out to area PCPs to emphasize the clinic's role as a partner in community health care. Most PCPs have longer wait times for appointments than they would like. PCPs who have established relationships with local CCCs can recommend the clinic to their patients for matters the patient feels cannot wait for the next available appointment. Part of the community health partnership should entail that the CCC and local providers have efficient and timely communication of patient data, so that, for instance, the outcome of the patient's CCC visit is relayed to the primary provider for more thorough follow-up. Thus, local providers should see the ability to refer patients for timely diagnosis and treatment as both good patient care and good customer service. A potentially frustrated and angry patient who could not be seen today instead appreciates the clinic for being an option and her doctor for recommending it.

CCCs can serve other partnership functions as well. There are times when a PCP will see a patient on a Friday and want next-day follow-up; the doctor can send the patient to the CCC the next day, knowing the visit outcome will be relayed back to the primary care office, and the clinic's most obvious community benefit is the availability of service outside of standard medical office hours. The clinic's evening and weekend hours meet the needs of people who feel they cannot wait until the next time their doctor's office is open, and after-hours service also diverts nonurgent care from local emergency departments.

Partnerships between retail-based health clinics and PCPs can vary from simple communication between collaborating physicians to signing formal affiliations with physician practices or health care systems. Formal affiliations can assist with recruitment of collaborating physicians and can include protocols to improve continuity of care through medical record sharing. There is no perfect relationship between CCCs and local PCPs, medical practices, and health systems. Part of the research a clinic operator conducts prior to launching the clinic should include relationship building with local providers.

NOTES

1. See National Council of State Boards of Nursing (https://www.ncsbn.org/index.htm) for the Nursing Model Act.
2. Compare TENN. COMP. R.&REGS 0880-6-.02 with TENN. COMP. R.&REGS 0880-2-.18

The Future of Convenient Care Clinics and Health Care Reform

JASON HWANG

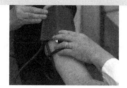

From their beginnings with the opening of the first QuickMedx stores in Minneapolis, convenient care clinics (CCCs) have become increasingly important providers of primary care for the general population. As health care reform in the United States promises significant change to the regulatory landscape, the future of CCCs lies in a continued evolution toward more sophisticated offerings while maintaining their core strength in convenience and efficiency. This evolution will provide attractive career paths for nurse practitioners and physician assistants, help lower the per-episode cost of care, and provide new avenues of growth for traditional health care providers such as hospitals and health care networks. As the industry evolves, practitioners and operators must take care to manage the host of opportunities and risks presented by patterns in disruptive innovation amid regulatory changes.

DISRUPTIVE INNOVATION THEORY

The disruptive innovation theory explains the process by which complicated, expensive products and services are transformed into simple, affordable ones. The theory's basic concepts are depicted in Figure 22.1, which charts the performance of a service or product over time. The solid line denotes the pace of improvement in products and services offered to customers as companies introduce newer and better products over time. Meanwhile, the dotted lines depict the improvements that customers are able to utilize; there are multiple dotted lines to represent the different tiers of customers within

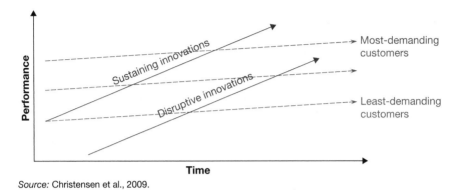

Source: Christensen et al., 2009.

Figure 22.1 ■ Model of disruptive innovation.

any given market, from the most demanding customers at the top to those at the bottom who are satisfied with very little. As the intersecting trajectories of the solid and dotted lines suggest, customers' needs in a given market application tend to be relatively stable over time, but companies typically improve their products at a much faster pace. Thus, products that at one point weren't good enough ultimately pack together more features and functions than customers need.

Occasionally, a different type of innovation emerges in an industry—a disruptive innovation. A disruptive innovation is not a breakthrough improvement. Instead of sustaining the traditional incumbent-player trajectory of improvement, the disruptor brings to market a product or service that is actually not as good as those of the leading companies, making it unattractive to existing customers. However, because they are simpler and more affordable, disruptive innovations attract nonconsumers who previously lacked the money or skill to buy and use the incumbent products. By competing on the basis of simplicity, affordability, and convenience, these disruptions are able to attract an entirely different group of customers. In contrast to traditional customers, these new users tend to be quite happy to have a low-end product because it is infinitely better than their only alternative, which is nothing at all. As the so-called low-end products naturally advance, they become good enough for even customers of the original products and eventually capture the broader market from incumbent players.

CCCs as Disruptive Innovation

An industry whose products or services are still so complicated and expensive that only people with a lot of money and expertise can own and use them is an industry that has not yet been disrupted—this is the situation in health care. However, as they do elsewhere, processes of disruption are beginning to appear in health care, where performance is generally related to the complexity of diagnosis and treatment of medical conditions. Within this context, medical advances

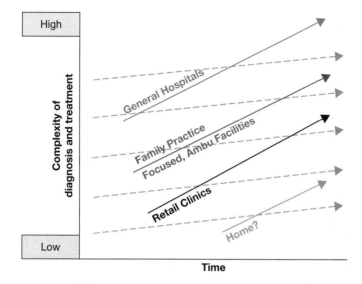

Figure 22.2 ■ Disruptive innovation in primary care delivery venues.

continuously raise the market's (patients') overall ability to enjoy more sophisticated care and better clinical outcomes. Specialist physicians and general hospitals reside on the cutting edge of medical innovations; conceptualizing, testing, and deploying ever-newer treatment procedures for more and more conditions. However, a large population of patients (low-income, uninsured, and those otherwise without access to health care) do not need the latest and greatest medical advances for their conditions. As a disruptive innovation, CCCs' limited offerings addressed only basic diagnoses and treatments and attracted patients who were looking for simple procedures with lower cost and higher convenience (see Figure 22.2).

CONVENIENT CARE AT A CROSSROADS

Like many disruptive business models that successfully captured a portion of the market previously dominated by a large incumbent, the convenient care industry finds itself facing a number of strategic decisions that will drive continued growth or lead to stagnation and decline. These strategic questions confronting the industry are:

- Should the clinics continue expanding their menu of offerings to patients?
- Should nurse practitioners and physician assistants continue to be the dominant providers in the clinics, or should other professionals begin to provide services?
- Should CCCs continue to compete with incumbent care providers through convenience or also compete on sophistication of diagnoses and treatments?

Expanded Offerings

We believe that CCCs must continue to expand their scope of service offerings to continue on their disruptive trajectory to traditional primary care delivery models. Continued expansion of offerings will create an attractive alternative career path for clinicians with a challenging and fulfilling work environment. Without progressing up the disruptive path, CCCs risk losing their ability to attract and retain practitioners, who could become increasingly frustrated with the rote and unfulfilling nature of treatments currently offered. Furthermore, unless the clinics can continue moving up the disruptive path, the industry risks being disrupted itself by alternative offerings from clinical pharmacists and at-home treatment by patients themselves. Although nurse practioners (NPs) and physician assistants (PAs) still face variable state-level regulations and are in many states subject to stringent restrictions on their practice, one potential step is to take advantage of telehealth technologies that permit distant physicians to interact with patients remotely, with providers on-site in the clinics acting as the "hands" of the physicians during the diagnosis and treatment. Because the technologies enable physicians to "see" more patients who would not have been theirs anyway, these physicians should be less resistant to allowing nurse practitioners and physician assistants to offer more sophisticated services in their presence in a telehealth context. As technological advances improve communications and simplify previously sophisticated tasks, we believe there will be more and more similar opportunities for CCCs to expand their offerings despite opposing forces (see Figure 22.3).

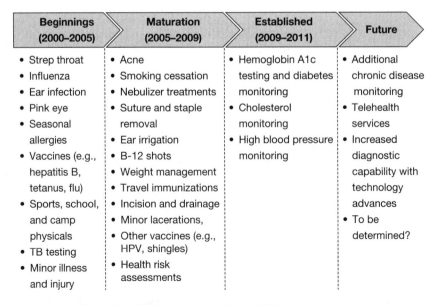

Beginnings (2000–2005)	Maturation (2005–2009)	Established (2009–2011)	Future
• Strep throat • Influenza • Ear infection • Pink eye • Seasonal allergies • Vaccines (e.g., hepatitis B, tetanus, flu) • Sports, school, and camp physicals • TB testing • Minor illness and injury	• Acne • Smoking cessation • Nebulizer treatments • Suture and staple removal • Ear irrigation • B-12 shots • Weight management • Travel immunizations • Incision and drainage • Minor lacerations, • Other vaccines (e.g., HPV, shingles) • Health risk assessments	• Hemoglobin A1c testing and diabetes monitoring • Cholesterol monitoring • High blood pressure monitoring	• Additional chronic disease monitoring • Telehealth services • Increased diagnostic capability with technology advances • To be determined?

Figure 22.3 ■ Sample of evolution of CCC service offerings.

Different Professionals in CCCs

Disruption of the primary care delivery model has occurred along both the venue of care delivery (e.g., hospital to primary care, primary care to clinic) and the professional who manages that care (e.g., physicians to nurse practitioners and physician assistants). We can predict future disruptive waves along both dimensions. As with the disruption in venue described earlier, there will likely be disruption in the type of professionals in the retail-based setting. Just as nurse practitioners and physician assistants are disrupting physicians by offering primary care independently, clinical pharmacists, who are already in the stores that host CCCs, have the potential to be disruptive by offering basic primary care services with greater convenience and lower cost. Rather than working to prevent this, providers in CCCs should embrace this trend to create opportunities to offer better services "up market" (see Figure 22.4).

Finally, both dimensions of disruption observed thus far still rest on existing equipment and infrastructure in hospitals and clinics. With advances in technology, patients' demand for better, more convenient primary care also portends new business models that offer even greater convenience—also known as infrastructure-independent services, such as house call services, telehealth, and wireless health models—that could be highly disruptive to CCCs. CCC operators who monitor these changes closely to take advantage of them, as with the telehealth example discussed in the previous section, rather than fall victim to them will be able to better manage the challenges to their business model that will surely arise.

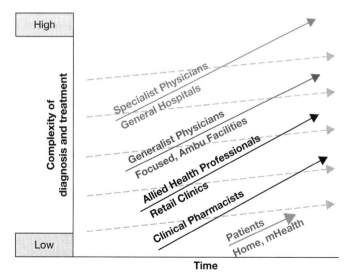

Figure 22.4 ■ Disruptive waves in primary care delivery professionals.

Value of Convenience

While it is critical for CCCs to continue advancing up market to expand the scope of services and provide fulfilling career paths for NPs, such expansion cannot come at the expense of convenience and efficiency for patients at the clinics. Although CCCs are increasingly becoming a component of existing health care delivery networks, their primary selling point over traditional primary care delivery models remains convenience. If the pursuit of up-market services leads to longer lines and wait times for patients, CCCs will find themselves competing more directly with traditional delivery venues in the sophistication of services—a battle traditional venues will surely win. The challenge to CCC operators, then, is to identify innovations in technology and operational practices that permit up-market services without sacrificing convenience.

Pathway to Growth

CCCs will undeniably play an increasingly large role in the U.S. health care system. Expanding care to formerly nonconsuming patients will increase the total cost of care for the population as a percentage of GDP; however, it will significantly lower the per-episode cost of care through the lower costs of retail-based care and the reduction in costly emergency visits for nonemergency care. CCCs further reduce burdens on the health care system by improving access to preventative care for nonconsumers.

Historically, CCCs grew by capturing the basic-services segment of the primary care delivery market by disrupting incumbent primary care clinics and general hospitals. As discussed earlier, the next engines of growth for the industry will be through expanding services up market, embracing other medical professionals such as pharmacists to participate in CCCs, and continuing to emphasize convenience. If current CCC operators (primarily pharmacies such as CVS Caremark and Walgreens) pursue these strategies, we predict they will continue to drive the majority of growth in the industry. In addition, another pathway to growth exists through large integrated players, for whom operating CCCs will in fact enable them to retain patients, expand service offerings, and compete with other large players deploying the clinics. Most important, operating CCCs will also allow large integrated players to push care delivery to the lowest-cost setting possible. Through linkages with hospital physicians, integrated health records, and inclusion in payer plans, CCCs have become a component of the mainstream health care system, with several consequences:

- More rapid expansion and adoption of the CCC concept (Only as long as the clinic is not a threat to more profitable businesses. For example, independently, a CCC should want to offer more services up-market, but a large system may not want this.)

- Exposure to a new wave of disruption from entrants catering to low-income and uninsured populations, for whom access to CCCs will also become limited if integrated players deploy them in markets aligned with their existing business models—middle-class to affluent populations with insurance coverage.

HEALTH CARE REFORM

Changes to the regulatory apparatus for health care delivery in the United States have been a subject of much debate and characterization, with constant flux in actual policy manifestations. Regardless of the latest enactments, several conditions will be critical to continued and effective growth for the convenient care industry.

Expanded Scope of Nursing Practice and Licensure

A regulatory environment that permits an expanded scope of nursing services is critical to enabling the up-market shift needed to drive further growth in CCCs. As with most health care regulations, the degrees to which local policies favor or hinder CCCs differ widely by state. In states such as Maryland and Arizona, NPs are licensed to provide primary care with minimal or no required involvement with physicians, while in Texas and Missouri, for example, physicians are required to be on-site and directly involved in primary care in some capacity. Similarly, state regulations vary as to how physician assistants and physicians must practice together, with certain states interpreting that relationship more permissively than others. There has been some clustering of CCCs in states with more permissive nurse practitioner regulations, and it is one of many factors clinic operators consider when locating a new clinic site. CCC proponents looking to gain access to more regions should look to the growing body of clinical and financial data from existing clinics as their strongest asset in presenting the case to regulators that NPs and PAs in CCCs are more than capable of delivering first-rate primary care at a lower cost. The promise of more care at a lower cost, in addition to the growing premium placed on convenient access to care in the face of the surge in covered patient population resulting from U.S. health care reform, will make CCCs increasingly attractive to regulators.

Several caveats exist for this approach. First, CCC operators and NPs must take extreme care in ensuring the cogency and integrity of clinical outcomes data from existing clinics—their strongest "arrow in the quiver" before regulators. As physicians and other incumbent "disruptees" are constantly vigilant for evidence pointing to reduced safety or quality of care at CCCs, any instance of misdiagnosis or accident will surely be found and used to help undermine the expansion of the clinics and scopes of their services. Second, NPs and PAs must take care to ensure their continued relevance in the most basic kinds of primary care even as the profession shifts up market. For instance, while trends such as the introduction of doctorate degrees in nursing practice point to upward shifts in the nursing profession, nurses risk appearing to abandon the basic primary care that forms the backbone of CCC offerings. Just as CCCs disrupted physicians who pursued increasingly sophisticated offerings away from primary care, any patient impression that NPs or PAs are also ignoring basic care will expose them to market disruption by "lower-end" providers such as pharmacists and providers of infrastructure-independent care.

Integrated Electronic Medical Records

Electronic medical or health records (EMRs or EHRs), the computerized recording, storage, and retrieval of patient medical data, are a key component of U.S. health care reform efforts. They are additionally a critical pathway for CCCs to gain more primacy within the primary care market through integration with established health care facilities. By ensuring that their internal IT systems are fully compatible and interactive with whatever EMR standards emerge, CCC operators will be able to be informed by and add to their patients' existing medical information, improving the quality of care and reducing the risk of misdiagnoses, mistreatments, and accidents. Furthermore, integrated databases between CCCs and other facilities, coupled with technological advances such as telemedicine, will further enable physicians to remotely supervise NPs and PAs in retail settings in localities with restrictive regulations and will facilitate growth of CCCs.

While designing and deploying standardized IT systems may face operational or technical challenges, the broader challenge before CCCs is the inherent reluctance of (and at times opposition from) established health care facilities such as hospitals and primary care clinics to share data with CCCs for fear of losing their patients. The onus is on CCCs to advance this integration through dialogue with other medical professions.

Access, Payment, and Patient Communication Reforms

Any reform that makes primary care more accessible to the general population will be conducive to CCCs' growth, primarily through increasing the patient base looking for primary care providers and the added premium on convenience that such growth in patient base naturally leads to. Aspirations towards universal coverage in the United States, if successful, will create a rapid increase in demand for primary care from previously uncovered groups. CCCs, with their ability to grow rapidly and cheaply compared with larger facilities, can capture much of this growth by being the first to address the increased demand, through more locations and expanded offerings. Furthermore, changes in employer and payer reimbursement policies that favor the use of CCCs (e.g., reimbursing 100% of CCC expenses versus 70% of primary care clinic or hospital expenses) will provide greater incentives for patients to use CCCs. While price-based incentives are a potential lever to attract more patients to CCCs, the clinics' relatively small price differential compared with traditional venues may not alone be sufficient to induce material change in patient behavior.

Finally, improvements in patient communication from health care providers will also support CCCs' growth. Despite clear differences in venue, convenience, and price between CCCs and traditional facilities, many patients are not yet aware of retail-based clinics as a viable option for their primary care needs. Efforts toward increasing transparency and awareness of primary care options, either through marketing campaigns or tools to aid consumers in making health care purchasing behaviors, will go a long way in supporting CCCs' growth amid health care reform changes.

CONCLUSION

Like many disruptive innovations, what began as humble outfits ridiculed by incumbent physicians—CCCs—irresistibly grew to capture increasing shares of the primary care delivery market through lower cost and greater convenience. Disruptive innovation theories predict continued growth and success from taking advantage of technological advances and promoting regulatory reforms that enable expanded service offerings for CCCs and carefully managed integration and collaboration with existing health care delivery networks. CCC clinicians, operators, and leaders who fully appreciate these opportunities and act accordingly will have the chance to play a significant role in bringing innovation to an infamously inefficient industry, improve the lives of patients, and create exciting opportunities for future generations of clinicians.

Appendix

Profiles of Clinic Operators

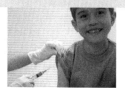

AURORA QUICKCARE CLINICS

"Convenient care clinics (CCCs) are a wonderful opportunity for nurse practitioners and physician assistants to pursue. The clinics give you the opportunity to practice in an autonomous manner in a unique setting. As the shortage of primary care providers grows, this is a perfect niche to help patients have easy, convenient access to health care in their time-starved daily lives."

Aurora Health Care opened the first Aurora QuickCare Clinics in 2004. Today, there are 13 Aurora QuickCare sites in Wisconsin, 10 public and 3 private. The clinics can be found in a variety of locations, including grocery stores, shopping malls, Aurora Pharmacies, and Walmart Supercenters.

What makes Aurora QuickCare Clinics are staffed by nurse practitioners and physician assistants who provide fast, convenient, and affordable diagnostic services and treatment for common family illnesses such as sore throat, ear infection, sinus infection, pink eye, mononucleosis, bladder infection, and bronchitis. In addition, Aurora QuickCare Clinics provide sport and camp physicals, cholesterol screenings, TB testing, and vaccinations, such as flu, meningitis, and tetanus. A typical visit takes just about 15 minutes, no appointment is necessary, and patients who require a prescription receive it before they leave.

What makes Aurora QuickCare Clinics unique is that it is one of the few clinic operators in the country that is part of a large, integrated health care system. Aurora includes a series of acute care hospitals, medical clinics, physician groups, retail pharmacy chains, home health agencies, behavioral health services, and hospice services. More information about Aurora QuickCare Clinics, including a list of locations, is available at www.Aurorahealthcare.org/quickcare.

BAPTIST EXPRESS CARE

Baptist Health, headquartered in Louisville, Kentucky, owns six acute care hospitals with more than 1,600 licensed beds in Corbin, La Grange, Lexington, Louisville, Paducah, and Richmond. Caring for Kentuckians since 1924, Baptist Health's mission is to exemplify its Christian heritage of providing quality health care services by enhancing the health of the people and the communities it serves.

Baptist Health opened its first Baptist Express Care clinic in 2009. Baptist Express Care provides fast, affordable access to basic health care services such as checkups, immunizations, screenings, and minor injuries. Located in select Walmart stores throughout Kentucky, Baptist Express Care is staffed by licensed, board-certified nurse practitioners ready to assist patients at a time that works best for their busy schedules.

Each clinic serves patients age 2 and older, and appointments are not necessary. Prices for services are posted clearly so that cost is always known before treatment. Baptist Express Care accepts cash and credit/debit cards as well as most major insurance plans.

Baptist Express Care clinics offer affordable options for treatment of minor illnesses and injuries as well as services such as cholesterol screening, blood sugar testing, vaccinations, drug screening, pregnancy testing, and TB testing.

Baptist Express Care clinics are located in Walmart stores in Berea, Corbin, Danville, LaGrange, Lexington, Louisville, Nicholasville, Paducah, Paris, Somerset, Williamsburg, and Winchester, Kentucky. For more information about Baptist Express Care, go to www.baptistexpresscare.com. To learn more about Baptist Health, please visit www.bhsi.com.

BAPTIST HEALTH SYSTEMS (MISSISSIPPI)

Baptist Health Systems is the parent company of Baptist Medical Center, the Mississippi Hospital for Restorative Care, Baptist Medical Center-Leake in Carthage, Mississippi, and a number of related health care services and programs. For over 100 years, Baptist Medical Center has served Mississippi and the surrounding states as a Christian-based, nonprofit comprehensive medical center. Visit Baptist on the web at www.mbhs.org.

BELLIN HEALTH—FASTCARE

"The convenient care industry can be a great opportunity for nurse practitioners and physician assistants from both a clinical and business perspective. Being involved with a health system that provides immediate access to health care for their patients, with a defined scope of service, creates high patient-satisfaction scores. This is due, in part, to creating convenient access for the patient and the opportunity for the provider to triage patients immediately into the primary care continuum of care. If a practitioner has a business interest and would like to manage personnel and manage clinics operated by the health system, opportunities can be available as well."

Bellin Health is a not-for-profit, integrated health care delivery system that has been servicing Northeast Wisconsin and Michigan's Upper Peninsula since 1908. Bellin Health is known for its emphasis on preventive health care and is the region's leader in cardiac, orthopedic, digestive, and mental health and primary care services. Bellin has been recognized several times as a 100 Top Hospital.

Bellin started the FastCare retail health clinic model in 2006. FastCare provides convenient and economical health care services for many basic health conditions. The clinic is staffed by nurse practitioners and physician assistants; the cost for a FastCare visit is $57 and can be billed to a person's insurance carrier. Among the types of conditions seen and treated at FastCare are sore throats, urinary tract infections, fevers, flu and colds, ear and sinus infections, upper respiratory infections, and allergies. There are 30 FastCare locations in 10 states, partnered with 20 health care systems located in retail settings. The clinics have convenient hours: Monday through Friday—8:30 a.m. to 8:30 p.m., Saturdays—8:30 a.m. to 5:00 p.m., Sundays—10:00 a.m. to 5:00 p.m., and holidays—10:00 a.m. to 2:00 p.m.

To ensure quality health services, Bellin built FastCare according to the guidelines for retail clinics as defined by the American Academy of Family Physicians, the American Academy of Pediatrics, and the American Medical Association. These include offering to send visit follow-up notes to PCPs, having a well-defined and limited scope of clinical services with evidence-based treatment plans, and having a system for referring patients to physicians when symptoms exceed the clinic's scope of services. In addition, prescriptions are filled quickly and transmitted electronically to each retailer's pharmacy or to a pharmacy of the patient's choice.

FastCare partners with local health care providers to establish CCCs in retail and grocery stores located throughout the country. More information about Bellin FastCare is available at www.bellinfastcare.com. For more information on Bellin Health see www.bellin.org.

GEISINGER CAREWORKS

"Geisinger Health System is dedicated to the expansion of the medical home model of care and population health. We utilize Careworks walk-in clinics in this model to expand access and lower costs. By positioning Careworks as an extension of primary care and sharing a common electronic medical record, we are able to create open access 7 days per week, 12 hours per day. This access dramatically lowers emergency room utilization and improves engagement and retention with primary care and the medical home. Not only are costs measurably lower, but outcomes improve due to early intervention and higher compliance rates."

Careworks walk-in clinics offer convenient, affordable health care provided by nurse practitioners and physician assistants from Geisinger Health System. Careworks diagnoses, treats, and writes prescriptions (when clinically appropriate) for common medical problems including colds and flu, allergies, insect bites, earaches, and sinus infections. The clinics also provide immunizations, screenings, and various wellness services. Some Careworks walk-in clinics also provide urgent care treatment of acute illnesses and minor injuries, helping patients avoid unnecessary emergency room visits. Services at these clinics also include x-ray, EKG, IV hydration, and phlebotomy. Careworks walk-in clinics are conveniently located and are open days, evenings, and weekends with no appointment necessary.

Careworks after-hours clinics: Providers at the after-hours clinics treat injuries or illnesses that require immediate treatment but may not be serious enough to warrant an ER visit. The after-hours clinics are open evenings and weekends and also do not require appointments.

Careworks on-site clinics: Careworks also operates on-site clinics that help reduce employer costs and increase productivity and employee satisfaction while improving access to quality care.

Careworks management services: In addition to successfully running its own clinics, Careworks also works with other hospitals and health systems across the country, offering consulting services and management solutions that enable health systems to capitalize on the opportunity to establish their own CCC networks.

HARRISON MEMORIAL HOSPITAL

Harrison Memorial Hospital, located in Cynthiana, Kentucky, is a community-owned, not-for-profit, 61-bed hospital, established in 1906. It offers a full range of services and an exceptional staff. HMH has an outstanding 18-member active staff, with more than 100 physicians on consulting staff. Harrison Memorial is considered by its peers a progressive entity in rural health.

THE HEALTHCARING CLINIC

The HealthCaring Clinic, a division of the HealthCaring Company, is a pioneer in consumer health care, led by a team with a proven track record. The HealthCaring Clinic offers walk-in medical care to patients 18 months and older with no appointment needed. The clinics are staffed by nurse practitioners who diagnose and treat a variety of common illnesses including strep throat, sinusitis, ear infections, bladder infections, and minor skin conditions. The HealthCaring Company also provides a wide range of wellness services including sports, school, camp, and pre-employment physicals; TB testing; and screenings, including cholesterol, blood sugar, and blood pressure. The clinic also offers prevention services such as flu, pneumonia, hepatitis, and tetanus vaccinations and provides prescriptions.

HERITAGE VALLEY HEALTH SYSTEMS

Heritage Valley Health System is a progressive community-based health care system located in southwestern Pennsylvania. In partnership with more than 425 physicians and nearly 4,100 employees, they offer a broad range of medical, surgical, and diagnostic services at hospitals, community satellite facilities, and in physician offices.

LAKEVIEW HEALTH/STILLWATER MEDICAL GROUP

What excites you about the CCC industry?

"I love working in an environment where people truly appreciate that we can offer high-quality medical exams in a walk-in setting and at an affordable price. We are open 362 days per year and make access to care more readily available during off hours and holidays when traditional primary care offices are closed."

What opportunities lie ahead for the industry?

"The retail setting is a portal of entry for many into the health care system. We see people from all walks of life, with all levels of experience 'in the system,' from the employed with full insurance coverage to the unemployed with none. Until access, cost, and quality issues are resolved for every American, there will be a place in the operational structure of care delivery for retail clinics. Expanding the scope of practice will necessitate even closer relationships with a patient's medical home, which is possible given the evolving technologies that have always been in place in retail clinics."

What makes it exciting to work in a CCC?

"Patients often dip their toes into the medical system by presenting to retail sites with conditions outside the retail scope of practice. Advanced practice providers (nurse practitioners and physician assistants) are uniquely positioned to triage these cases to the appropriate level of care. This necessitates keeping skills sharp, a differential diagnosis, and excellent communication skills with a network of ancillary community providers and facilities.

In a world where many health care concerns become compartmentalized and off-loaded to other departments to be addressed at other visits, the retail visit allows a provider the opportunity to do patient teaching in a nontraditional setting in which the patient may be more receptive to teaching and health education."

Lakeview Health is an integrated, nonprofit clinic and hospital system serving a population of more than 250,000 residents in the eastern Twin Cities' metro area and western Wisconsin. Lakeview Health includes a multispecialty physician/provider group (Stillwater Medical Group [SMG]), an acute care hospital, and a foundation that raises funds to advance the mission of Lakeview Health. The system has garnered national and local acclaim for achievements in quality, patient satisfaction, and orthopedic surgery. Lakeview Health is a member of the HealthPartners family of care.

SMG is certified by the Minnesota Department of Health as a health care home. SMG employs 310 individuals, totaling 247.32 FTEs. Approximately 39% of employees are full time, 52% are part time, and 9% are casual. The average length of service for all SMG employees is 6.53 years.

Facilities include a 110,595-square-foot main and specialty clinic and a 33,564-square-foot OB/GYN clinic, both in Stillwater, and a 13,042-square-foot clinic in Somerset, Wisconsin. SMG staffs and operates a CCC located inside Walmart in Oak Park Heights, Minnesota. A community pharmacy is located at the Curve Crest Clinic facility. SMG's physicians and staff work together to address primary and specialty care needs that include family medicine, internal medicine, OB/GYN, pediatrics and adolescent medicine, allergy, audiology, cardiology, dermatology, emergency medicine, foot and ankle surgery, gastroenterology, geriatrics, neurology, otolaryngology, oncology, physical therapy, sports medicine, urology, and occupational health.

LINDORA HEALTH CLINICS

What excites you about the CCC industry?

"At Lindora, we've long believed that CCCs are the perfect venue for treating chronic conditions, especially those that involve a change in lifestyle. By definition, the clinics are accessible and such easy accessibility removes a barrier for compliance and therefore promotes adherence and enhanced outcome."

What opportunities lie ahead for the industry?

"We see CCCs playing a much more significant role in patient-centered medicine, particularly in the areas of lifestyle medicine such as the treatment of obesity, diabetes, hypertension, and asthma. As people's lives seem to become busier, accessibility and convenience become increasingly more important. When people can handle a medical appointment, buy groceries or a new sweater, and pick up a prescription all in one location, it eliminates one of the obstacles in taking care of oneself and one's family."

What makes it exciting to work in a CCC?

"Our Lindora health clinic staff loves the variety and spontaneity that working in a CCC provides. One minute, they're sharing in the joy of a patient who has just hit a weight loss milestone on our program. An hour later, they may be examining a patient who is visiting from out of town and has developed strep throat. Our team thrives on the challenge of making important decisions on the spot and helping real people deal with real health issues. They also love the independence and autonomy of essentially running their own clinic. There is no typical day, and that is what makes it so interesting."

Lindora Health Clinics were the first in-store clinics in America to offer medically supervised weight control treatment in addition to nonemergency medical care. The first Lindora Health Clinics were opened in 2006 in a partnership with Rite Aid, and the clinics are promoted as "The most convenient way to feel *and* look better." There are currently seven Lindora Health Clinic locations throughout Southern California, and more than 400 Rite Aid stores also carry a selection of Lindora's most popular program-compliant nutritional products.

Lindora was founded in 1971 by Marshall Stamper, MD, and operates 35 Southern California clinics specializing in weight management and obesity medicine, in addition to their seven CCCs. Long recognized as the gold standard in medically supervised weight management, their Lean for Life® program combines diet, moderate exercise, and motivational support to help patients lose weight and learn to successfully keep it off while improving their metabolic fitness.

Lindora Health Clinics are staffed by nurse practitioners, physician's assistants, and additional allied health professionals. All services are offered on a walk-in basis. In addition to offering the Lindora weight loss program, Lindora Health Clinics treat a wide range of nonemergency acute care conditions. Diagnostic screenings, sports physical examinations, and a variety of immunizations are also offered.

THE LITTLE CLINIC

"Just as many industries have had to evolve to meet consumer demand, the outpatient health care industry is experiencing similar change. Banks were forced to move from their nine to three mentalities to 24-hour ATMs and even online banking if they wanted to stay in business. Travel agents have become sparse with the advent of 'dot com' alternatives. In health care, change has always been slow and often contentious. A hundred years ago, the AMA declared group practice unethical; now it is largely the norm and even has its own representative section within the AMA house of delegates. Outpatient surgery centers were touted by many in years past as unsafe, and they are now commonplace, accredited, and probably safer than inpatient facilities with regard to facility-acquired infections. The convenient care industry has faced significant criticism from traditional physician organizations such as the AMA, AAFP, and AAP, yet the consumer uptake continues to grow rapidly, and well-respected academic medical centers and medical groups have come to see the value in affiliating with convenient care companies to serve as care entry portals, post–hospital discharge follow-ups, after-hours routine care, and monitoring of chronic care; in essence, to be an integral part of the patient-centered medical home model. They do this because the quality of care has been established, the cost-effectiveness is clear, and the likelihood of patient compliance is improved when convenience of time and place is offered."

Founded in 2003 and headquartered in Nashville, Tennessee, The Little Clinic is a pioneer in customer-focused health care with a mission to provide convenient, affordable health care, and wellness education. A wholly owned subsidiary of the Kroger Company The Little Clinic health care clinics are currently located inside select Kroger stores in Georgia, Kentucky, Tennessee, and Ohio; King Soopers in Colorado; and Fry's Food Stores in Arizona. The Little Clinic earned accreditation by The Joint Commission and has been awarded its Gold Seal of Approval®. Visit The Little Clinic online at www.thelittleclinic.com, www.facebook.com/thelittleclinic, and www.thelittleclinic.blogspot.com.

MEDPOINT EXPRESS

"MEDPOINT express is very excited about the future of the convenient care industry as we believe it is poised for incredible growth and will play an increasing role as a low-cost access point for patients that is an extension of the patient-centered medical home. Future partnership opportunities with health systems and payers should also greatly enhance the industry's prominence as a key part of the health care continuum."

MEDPOINT express is a subsidiary of Memorial Health System of South Bend, Indiana and has been offering convenient and cost-effective care for the treatment of minor health conditions since 2005, when it opened the first medical clinic located inside a Walmart Superstore in August 2005. MEDPOINT express brings quality health care in step with busy lives by offering convenient medical services right where today's busy consumers live, work, shop, and play. Its nurse practitioners perform physical examinations and treat common illnesses, such as fevers, rashes, ear infections, coughs, and flu for anyone age 2 or older. MEDPOINT express operates four clinics and accepts most insurance. Clinics are located in Martin's Supermarkets and Walmart Superstores in northern Indiana. For more information on the services offered, pricing, hours, and locations, visit www.medpointexpress.com or call 1-800-635-5516.

MILWAUKEE HEALTH SERVICES

Milwaukee Health Services, Inc. (MHSI) is a federally qualified health center (FQHC) providing medical services to approximately 32,000 vulnerable and underserved patients each year.

In 2009, MHSI gained distinction among the national FQHCs by being the first to open a retail-based health clinic. At that time, MHSI began a partnership with Centene Corporation, the parent company of Managed Health Services—a major health management organization (HMO) provider—to open the MHS CCC inside the Midtown Piggly Wiggly grocery store.

The Midtown Piggly Wiggly is owned and operated by the Martin family, which allowed MHSI the opportunity to partner with a store in a geographical area that has a high concentration of Medicaid recipients as well as the underserved and uninsured.

The MHS CCC is owned and operated by MHSI. As is true with MHSI's two main clinics, this site offers affordable and quality health care. Various acute care services, vaccines, and screenings are also provided. The MHS CCC offers a very similar scope of services to those provided at retail care clinics operated by pharmacies and hospitals.

Services at the MHS CCC are provided by a nurse practitioner or physician assistant, with additional support by medical assistants. The NPs and PAs are trained, board-certified clinicians who can provide acute care and write prescriptions, not including pain management medication, at the MHS CCC. Retail-based health clinics are not intended to be replacements for primary care physicians, but many customers, as noted, do not have a medical home. Unlike many CCCs, MHSI is able to link its CCC patients to primary care providers within the organization's main clinics if they do not already have a medical home.

Services available at the MHS CCC include asthma and bronchitis; seasonal allergies; sinus infections; flu and common cold; cold sores; migraines; heartburn and reflux; bladder infections; ear infections; diarrhea, nausea and vomiting; pink eye, styes, and other eye-related infections; insect bites; poison ivy, acne, eczema, ringworm, and other skin rashes; and school and sports physicals.

The mission of MHSI is to provide accessible, high-quality primary and related health care services to Milwaukee residents, with the continuing emphasis on the medically underserved.

MINUTECLINIC

MinuteClinic is a division of CVS Caremark Corporation, the largest pharmacy health care provider in the United States. MinuteClinic launched the first retail-based medical clinics in the United States in 2000 and is the largest CCC provider, with approximately 600 locations in 25 states and the District of Columbia. By creating a health care delivery model that responds to consumer demand, MinuteClinic makes access to high-quality medical treatment easier for more Americans. Nationally, the company has generated more than 13 million patient visits, with a 95% customer satisfaction rating.

MinuteClinic is the only retail health care provider to receive three consecutive accreditations from The Joint Commission, the national evaluation and certifying agency for nearly 15,000 health care organizations and programs in the United States. For more information, visit www. MinuteClinic.com.

NORTH MISSISSIPPI MEDICAL CLINICS

What excites you about the CCC industry?

"We are excited that we have the opportunity to provide convenient, cost-effective, and quality health care for the people in our region. We know that access to care continues to be a problem in so many rural areas, and we feel that the CCC concept is a solution to this ongoing problem. We are able to offer care at a cost that is transparent to the patient and access that is quick and convenient."

What opportunities lie ahead for the industry?

"We look forward to expanding our CCC industry into new locations in our service area."

What makes it exciting to work in a CCC?

"One of our nurse practitioners, says, 'My job in a convenient care clinic is very exciting. Our staff works as a team, building lasting relationships with our patients while providing quality care in a compassionate manner. The clinic is fast paced, and the enthusiasm of our patients for the quick and convenient care is contagious!'"

North Mississippi Health Services is a diversified regional health care organization that serves 24 counties in north Mississippi and northwest Alabama from headquarters in Tupelo, Mississippi. The North Mississippi Medical Center (NMHS) organization covers a broad range of acute diagnostic and therapeutic services, offered through North Mississippi Medical Center in Tupelo; a community hospital system with locations in Eupora, Iuka, Pontotoc, and West Point, Mississippi, and Hamilton, Alabama; North Mississippi Medical Clinics, a regional network of more than 30 primary and specialty clinics; and nursing homes. NMHS offers a comprehensive portfolio of managed care plans.

North Mississippi also offers two CCCs, in Oxford and Columbus, both located in Walmarts. The clinics diagnose and treat a number of illnesses and minor injuries and also offer vaccinations and preparticipation physical examinations.

Educational programs and early intervention are important aspects of their services, but their main focus is to provide convenient access to quality health care. NMHS works to achieve its corporate mission to improve the health of the people of this region by providing conveniently accessible, cost-effective health care of the highest quality.

REDICLINIC

RediClinic has given consumers easy access to high-quality, affordable health care since 1989. The company currently operates 30 clinics inside H-E-B grocery stores in Houston, Austin, and San Antonio, Texas and has successfully treated more than 1,000,000 patients since opening its first in-store clinic in 2005. In addition to treating common medical conditions, RediClinics provide a broad range of preventive services, including medical tests, immunizations, and basic physical examinations, and the company's Weigh Forward program is the nation's only comprehensive, medically supervised weight management program offered in a grocery store. For more information on clinic locations, hours of operation, services, and prices, visit www.rediclinic.com.

TAKE CARE HEALTH SYSTEMS

Take Care Health Systems, a subsidiary of Walgreens, is a network of health and wellness companies committed to providing affordable, high-quality health care for families and employees.

Take Care Health Systems—the parent of Take Care Consumer Solutions and Take Care Employer Solutions—combines best practices in health and wellness for both families and employees under one convenient roof.

"Nursing and nursing leadership have played a critical role in the creation, scalability, and sustainability of the convenient care industry. As the first chief nurse practitioner officer in the industry, a founding officer of Take Care Health Systems, and a founding member of the Convenient Care Association, I have personally seen this industry grow from a novel idea to a reality to a permanent access point into the health care system that is loved by patients and respected by the health care community.

At the beginning, it was nurse practitioners who were willing to take the risk and work in these nontraditional settings seeing patients. The nurse practioners were pioneers, risk takers, and problem solvers who every day saw the issues patients were facing and knew better than most that the current traditional system was failing them. Nurse practitioners on the front line and nursing leadership on the ground in the communities being served led in the development of and adherence to quality and safety standards for the industry. Nursing leaders functioning as both clinical and business leaders pushed for certification processes; developed processes, procedures, and standardization around patient delivery; and precisely delivered, to millions of patients, evidence-based quality care that exceeded national standards.

As an industry spotlighting the care delivered in an autonomous setting by highly educated and trained providers, we needed to collect data to substantiate that we were delivering quality care and an exceptional patient experience. Today, the industry and the care that nurse practioners deliver are recognized as sustainable, worthwhile options that provide care that is not only of quality equal to or better than that of other traditional settings but that also exceeds the patients' expectations. Patients truly love the nurse practitioners and their ability to take care of them.

If the industry is to continue to grow in number of clinics, scope of services, and partnerships to meet the health care needs of the future, it will be important to continue to look at and evaluate the roles that NPs will play in care delivery, education, management, and leadership. The ability to truly 'take care' of patients will depend on having the right structure, resources, and support for this invaluable workforce."

Sandra Festa Ryan, RN, MSN, CPNP, FAANP
Chief Nurse Practitioner Officer, Take Care Health Systems

Take Care Consumer Solutions manages more than 350 Take Care Clinics at select Walgreens throughout the country. Each clinic is open 7 days a week to provide easy, affordable access to high-quality health care for adults and children. Patient care at Take Care Clinics is provided by Take Care Health Services, an independently owned state professional corporation.

Take Care Employer Solutions provides work-site-based health and wellness services. This group manages primary care, wellness, and occupational health centers at nearly 370 employer campuses across the country.

All combined, Take Care Health Systems manages more than 700 work-site health centers and retail-based clinics.

TARGET CLINIC

Target Clinic was introduced in 2006 to provide guests with access to quality, convenient, and affordable health care services. Target Clinic offers guests more than 60 services for minor illnesses and injuries, skin treatments, vaccinations, tests, and screenings. Target Clinic accepts most insurance plans and offers walk-in medical care 7 days a week, including nights and weekends with no appointment needed. By the end of 2013, Target will be operating nearly 70 Target Clinics in select states nationwide. For information on Target Clinic locations or services, visit Target.com/Clinics.

Minneapolis-based Target Corporation serves people at 1,808 stores—1,784 in the United States and 24 in Canada—and at Target.com. Since 1946, Target has given 5% of its profit through community grants and programs. Today, that giving equals more than $4 million a week.

SUTTER EXPRESS CARE (SUTTER HEALTH)

What excites you about the CCC industry?

"Convenient care is really an additional access for patients in need. The service provides care to many uninsured or underinsured patients and will continue to evolve to fill the gap between a physician's office, the hospital, the emergency department, and the patient—the gap will only grow with health reform and we have an important role to play to foster continuity while providing convenient access."

What opportunities lie ahead for the industry?

"Programs that patients find difficult to access—that will depend on the community in many ways. Immunizations, health maintenance, programmatic offerings like weight loss, and participation in chronic disease management by being a data collection point for disease management programs up to and including managing mild- to moderate-severity chronic illnesses. We will need to continue to look for the gaps to fill in total care for people."

What makes it exciting to work in a CCC?

"The biggest enticement is the independence of the environment. This becomes a clinician's clinic; they own it and they take pride in their work and their role."

Serving more than 100 Northern California cities and towns, Sutter Health offers a vast system of doctors, not-for-profit hospitals, and other health care service providers who share resources and expertise to advance health care quality and access. The Sutter Medical Network includes many of California's top-performing, highest quality (as measured annually by the Integrated Healthcare Association) physician organizations as well as the Sutter Express Care clinics, walk-in medical clinics located inside select Rite Aid stores next to the pharmacy.

Sutter Express Care clinics accept many health plans and have a flat fee of $69 for most services. Visits are quick and no appointments are necessary. The clinics are open 7 days a week, and each clinic is staffed by clinicians who have advanced training to diagnose and prescribe medication for common family illnesses such as strep throat; eye, ear, and sinus infections; and bronchitis. In total, the clinics treat over 36 common ailments in addition to providing vaccinations, sports physicals, preventive health screenings, and a popular weight loss program.

References

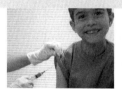

2011 ENA Emergency Nursing Resources Development Committee. (2011). Non-invasive temperature measurement in the emergency department. Retrieved from http://www.ena.org/IENR/ENR/Documents/TemperatureMeasurementENR.pdf

Accredidation Commission for Health Care. (2012). ACHC history. http://www.achc.org/aboutachc/history

Agency for Healthcare Research and Quality. (2011). Expenses and characteristics of physician visits in different ambulatory care settings, 2008. Retrieved from http://meps.ahrq.gov/mepsweb/data_files/publications/st318/stat318.pdf

Agency for Healthcare Research and Quality. (2012). National quality measures clearinghouse. Retrieved from http://www.qualitymeasures.ahrq.gov/tutorial/index.aspx

American Academy of Pain Management. (n.d.). Pain issues: Pain is an epidemic. Retrieved from http://aapainmanage.org/literature/Articles/PainAnEpidemic.pdf

American College of Obstetricians and Gynecologists. (2008). ACOG practice bulletin no. 91: Treatment of urinary tract infections in nonpregnant women. *Obstetrics and Gynecology, 111*, 785–794.

American Geriatrics Society 2012 Beers Criteria Update Expert Panel. (2012). American Geriatrics Society updated beers criteria for potentially inappropriate medication use in older adults. *Journal of the American Geriatrics Society, 60*(4), 616–631. doi:10.1111/j.1532-5415.2012.03923.x

American Heart Association. (n.d.) Hypertensive Crisis. Last updated April 4, 2012. Retrieved from http://www.heart.org/HEARTORG/Conditions/HighBloodPressure/AboutHighBloodPressure/Hypertensive-Crisis_UCM_301782_Article.jsp

Antibiotics for strep throat (streptococcal pharyngitis). *eMedExpert*. Last modified May 17, 2011. Retrieved from http://www.emedexpert.com/conditions/strep-throat.shtml

Aring, A. M., & Chan, M. M. (2011). Acute rhinosinusitis in adults. *American Family Physician, 83*, 1057–1063.

Arruda, E., Pitkaranta, A., Witek, T., Jr., Doyle, C. A., & Hayden, F. G. (1997). Frequency and natural history of rhinovirus infections in adults during autumn. *Journal of Clinical Microbiology, 35*, 2864–2868.

Ashwood, J. S., Reid, R. O., Setodji, C. M., Weber, E., Gaynor, M., & Mehrotra, A. (2011). Trends in retail clinic use among the commercially insured. *The American Journal of Managed Care, 17*, e443–e448.

Aung, K. (2011, September 26). Viral pharyngitis. *Medscape.* Retrieved from http://emedicine.medscape.com/article/225362-overview

Beach, J. (2008). Sinusitis. In T. Buttaro, J. Trybulski, P. P. Bailey, & J. Sandberg-Cook (Eds.), *Primary care: A collaborative practice* (3rd ed., pp. 365–368). St. Louis, MO: Mosby, Inc.

Bent, S., Nallamothu, B. K., Simel, D. L., Fihn, S. D., & Saint, S. (2002). Does this woman have an acute uncomplicated urinary tract infection? *Journal of the American Medical Association, 287,* 2701–2710. doi:10.1001/jama.287.20.2701

Berardi, R. R. (2009). *Handbook of nonprescription drugs: An interactive approach to self-care* (16th ed.). Washington, DC: American Pharamcists Association.

Bernhardt, D. T., & Roberts, W. O. (Eds.). (2010). *Preparticipation physical examination* (4th ed.). Elk Grove Village, IL: American Academy of Pediatrics.

Bisno, A., Gerber, M. A., Gwaltney J. M., Jr., Kaplan, E. L., & Schwartz, R. H. (2002). Practice guidelines for the diagnosis and management of group A streptococcal pharyngitis. *Clinical Infectious Diseases, 35,* 113.

Bolser, D. C. (2006). Cough suppressant and pharmacologic protussive therapy: ACCP evidence-based clinical practice guidelines. *Chest, 129*(1_suppl), 238S–249S.

Bono, M. (2011, March 29). Mycoplasma pneumonia. *Medscape.* Retrieved from http://emedicine.medscape.com/article/1941994-overview

Bradley, J. G., & Davis, K. A. (2003). Orthostatic hypotension. *American Family Physician, 68,* 2393–2399. Retrieved from http://nestor.orpha.net/AFHOI/upload/file/radley(2003).pdf

Bramam, S. S. (2006). Chronic cough due to acute bronchitis: ACCP evidence-based clinical practice guidelines. *CHEST, 129*(Suppl. 1), 95S–103S, 104S–115S.

Bremnor, J. D., & Sadovsky, R. (2002). Evaluation of dysuria in adults. *American Family Physician, 65,* 1589–1596.

Bridges, E., & Thomas, K. (2009). Ask the experts. Noninvasive measurement of body temperature in critically ill patients. *Critical Care Nurse, 29,* 94–97. doi:10.4037/ccn2009132

Brown, M. (2012). AAFP, USPSTF recommend screening all adults for obesity, offering some patients lifestyle intervention. Retrieved from http://www.aafp.org/online/en/home/publications/news/news-now/health-of-the-public/20120704obesityrecs.html

Brusch, J. (2012, February 21). Urinary tract infection in males: Treatment and management. *Medscape.* Retrieved from http://emedicine.medscape.com/article/231574-treatment#aw2aab6b5b3

Campbell, M., & Super, E. (2003, Spring). Histamine. *Davidson University Biology 307: Immunology.* Retrieved from http://www.bio.davidson.edu/Courses/Immunology/Students/Spring2003/Super/home.html

Cefalu, C. (2011). Theories and mechanisms of aging. *Clinics in Geriatric Medicine, 27,* 491–506.

Centers for Disease Control and Prevention. (2011, December). Retrieved November 8, 2011, from http://www.cdc.gov

Centers for Disease Control and Prevention. (2012, July 27). *Conjunctivitis.* Retrieved from http://www.cdc.gov/conjunctivitis/clinical.html

Chapman, R. S., Henderson, F. W., Clyde, W. A., Jr., Collier, A. M., & Denny, F. W. (1981). The epidemiology of tracheobronchitis in pediatric practice. *American Journal of Epidemiology, 114,* 786–797.

Cherry, D. K., Burt, C. W., & Woodwell, D. A. (2011, July 17). *National Ambulatory Medical Care Survey 1999* (DHHS Publication No. [PHS] 2001-125001-0383). Atlanta, GA: Centers for Disease Control and Prevention National Center for Health Statistics.

Chiappini, E., Venturini, E., Principi, N., Longhi, R., Tovo, P. A., Becherucci, P., ... de Martino, M. (2012). Update of the 2009 Italian society guidelines about management of fever in children (Electronic version). *Clinical Therapeutics, 34*(7), 1648–1653.

Chobanian, A. V., Bakris, G. L., Black, H. R., Cushman, W. C., Green, L. A., Izzo, J. L., Jr., ... National High Blood Pressure Education Program Coordinating Committee. (2003). Seventh report of the joint national committee on prevention, detection, evaluation, and treatment of high blood pressure. *Hypertension, 42*, 1206–1252. doi:10.1161/01.HYP.0000107251.49515.c2

Chow, A. W., Benninger, M. S., Brook, I., Brozek, J. L., Goldstein, E. J. C., Hicks, L. A., ... File, T. M., Jr. (2012). IDSA clinical practice guideline for acute bacterial rhinosinusitis in children and adults. *Clinical Infectious Diseases, 54*, e72–e112. doi:10.1093/cid/cir1043

Christensen, C., Grossman, J., & Hwang, J. (2009). *The innovator's prescription: A disruptive solution for health care*. New York, NY: McGraw-Hill.

Clarke, P. (2011, May 21). FDA encourages pediatric information on drug labeling. Retrieved from http://www.fda.gov/Drugs/ResourcesForYou/SpecialFeatures/ucm254072.htm

Consumer Healthcare Products Association. (2012) OTC sales by category—2008-2011. Retrieved from http://www.chpa-info.org/pressroom/Sales_Category.aspx

Cronau, H. K., Kankanala, R. R., & Mauger, T. (2010). Diagnosis and management of red eye. *American Family Physician, 81*, 37–44.

Cunha, J. P. (2012, April 11). High blood pressure (hypertension). *MedicineNet*. Retrieved from http://www.medicinenet.com/high_blood_pressure/article.htm

Delzell, J. E., Jr., & Lefevre, M. L. (2000). Urinary tract infections during pregnancy. *American Family Physician, 61*, 713–720.

Donaldson, M., Yordy, K., & Vanselow, N. (Eds.). (1994). *Defining primary care: An interim report* (p. 1). Washington, DC: The National Academies Press.

Egan, B. M., Zhao, Y., & Axon, N. (2010). U.S. trends in prevalence, awareness, treatment, and control of hypertension, 1988-2008. *Journal of the American Medical Association, 303*, 2043–2050. doi:10.1001/jama.(2010).650

Eloy, P., Poirrier, A. L., De Dorlodot, C., Van Zele, T., Watelet, J. B., & Bertrand, B. (2011). Actual concepts in rhinosinusitis: A review of clinical presentations, inflammatory pathways, cytokine profiles, remodeling, and management. *Current Allergy Asthma Respiratory, 11*, 146–162. doi:10.1007/s11882-011-0180-0

Ely, J. W., Hansen, M. R., & Clark, E. C. (2008). Diagnosis of ear pain. *American Family Physician, 77*, 621–628.

Feiner, J. R., Severinghaus, J. W., & Bickler, P. E. (2007). Dark skin decreases the accuracy of pulse oximeters at low oxygen saturation: The effects of oximeter probe type and gender. *Anesthesia and Analgesia, 105*, S18–S23. doi:10.1213/01.ane.0000285988.35174.d9

Ference, J. D., & Last, A. R. (2009). Choosing topical corticosteroids. *American Family Physician, 79*, 135–140.

Ferguson, B. J., Narita, M., Yu, V. L., Wagener, M. M., & Gwaltney, J. M., Jr. (2012). Prospective observational study of chronic rhinosinusitis: Environmental triggers and antibiotic implications. *Clinical Infectious Diseases, 54*, 62–68. doi: 10.1093/cid/cir747

File, T. (2012, September 19). Acute bronchitis in adults. *UpToDate*. Retrieved from http://www.uptodate.com/contents/acute-bronchitis-in-adults?source=see_link

Finkelstein, J. A., Christiansen, C. L., & Platt, R. (2000). Fever in pediatric primary care: Occurrence, management and outcomes (Electronic version). *Pediatrics, 105*, 260–266.

Fleisher, G. (2012, January 31). Evaluation of dysuria in children. *UpToDate*. Retrieved from http://www.uptodate.com/contents/evaluation-of-dysuria-in-children?source=search_result&search=dysuria&selectedTitle=1%7E150

Fleisher, G. (2012, May 9). Evaluation of sore throat in children. *UpToDate*. Retrieved from http://www.uptodate.com/contents/evaluation-of-sore-throat-in-children

Fokkens, W., Lund, V., & Mullol, J. (2007). EP3OS 2007: European position paper on rhinosinusitis and nasal polyps 2007. A summary for otorhinolaryngologists. *Rhinology, 45*, 97.

Food and Drug Administration. (2009, May 28). OTC drug facts label. Retrieved from http://www.fda.gov/Drugs/ResourcesForYou/Consumers/ucm143551.htm

Food and Drug Administration. (2013, March 12). http://www.fda.gov/Drugs/DrugSafety/ucm341822.htm

Gerber, M. A. (1989). Comparison of throat cultures and rapid strep tests for diagnosis of streptococcal pharyngitis. *The Pediatric Infectious Disease Journal, 8*, 820–824.

Giese, E. A., O'Connor, F. G., Brennan, F. H., Jr., Depenbrock, P. J., & Oriscello, R. G. (2007). The athletic preparticipation evaluation: Cardiovascular assessment. *American Family Physician, 75*, 1008–1014.

Gilbert, D. N., Moellering, R., Jr., Eliopoulos, G. M., & Saag, G. M. (2011). *The sanford guide to antimicrobial therapy 2011* (41st ed.). Sperryville, VA: Antimicrobial Therapy Inc.

Goguen, L. A. (2011, September 13). External otitis: Pathogenesis, clinical features, and diagnosis. *UpToDate*. Retrieved from http://www.uptodate.com/contents/external-otitis-pathogenesis-clinical-features-and-diagnosis

Goguen, L. A. (2012, April 12). External otitis: Treatment. *UpToDate*. Retrieved from http://www.uptodate.com/contents/external-otitis-treatment

Gonzales, R., Bartlett, J. G., Besser, R. E., Hickner, J. H., Hoffman, J. R., & Sande, M. A. (2001). Principles of appropriate antibiotic use for treatment of nonspecific upper respiratory tract infections in adults: background. *Annals of Internal Medicine, 134*, 490–494.

Gonzales, R., Bartlett, J. G., Besser, R. E., Cooper, R., Hickner, J., Hoffman, J., & Sande, M. (2001). Principles of appropriate antibiotic use for treatment of uncomplicated acute bronchitis: Background. *Annals of Internal Medicine, 134*, 521–529.

Goodhue, C. J., & Brady, M. A. (2004). Atopic and rheumatic disorders. In C. E. Burns, A. M. Dunn, M. A. Brady, N. B. Starr, & C. G. Blosser (Eds.), *Pediatric primary care: A handbook for nurse practitioners* (3rd ed., pp. 820–822). St. Louis, MO: Saunders.

Goroll, A. H., & Mulley, A. (Eds.) (2006). *Primary care medicine: Office evaluation and management of the adult patient* (5th ed.). Philadelphia, PA: Lippincott, Williams and Wilkins.

Gosselin, B. (2012, August 21). Peritonsillar abscess. *Medscape*. Retrieved from http://www.emedicine.medscape.com/article/194863-overview

Graneto, J. (2011, November 8). Emergent management of pediatric patients with fever. *Medscape*. Retrieved from http://emedicine.medscape.com/article/801598-overview

Greene, P. (2000). Pearls for practice: Recognizing young people at risk for sudden cardiac death in preparticipation sports physicals. *Journal of the American Academy of Nurse Practitioners, 12*, 11–14. doi:10.1111/j.1745-7599.2000.tb00275.x

Grijalva, C. G., Nuorti, J. P., & Griffin, M. R. (2009). Antibiotic prescription rates for acute respiratory tract infections in U.S. ambulatory settings. *Journal of the American Medical Association, 302*, 758–766. doi:10.1001/jama.2009.1163

Gunder, L. M., & Lanning, L. C. (2010). The sports physical. *Clinician Reviews/Convenient Care, 3*, 3–8.

Gupta, K., Hooton, T. M., Naber, K. G., Wullt, B., Colgan, R., Miller, L. G., … Soper, D. E. (2011). International clinical practice guidelines for the treatment of acute uncomplicated cystitis and pylonephritis in women: A 2010 update by the infectious disease society of America and the European society for microbiology and infectious diseases. *Clinical Infectious Diseases, 52*, e103–e120.

Haas, W., Pillar, C. M., Torres, M., Morris, T. W., & Sahm, D. F. (2011). Monitoring antibiotic resistance in ocular microorganisms: Results from the antibiotic resistance in ocular microorganisms (armor) 2009 surveillance study. *American Journal of Ophthalmology, 152*, 567–574.

Habif, T. P. (2004). Clinical dermatology: A color guide to diagnosis and therapy (4th ed.). Philadelphia, PA: Mosby.

Habif, T. P., Campbell, J. L., Jr., Chapman, M. S., Dinulos, J. G. H., & Zug, K. A. (2006). *Dermatology*. Philadelphia, PA: Mosby.

Halsey, E. (2012, January 11). Bacterial pharyngitis. *UpToDate*. Retrieved from http://emedicine.medscape.com/article/225243-overview

Hansen-Turton, T., Ridgway, C., Ryan, S. F., & Nash, D. B. (2009). Convenient care clinics: The future of accessible health care—The formation years 2006-2008. *Population Health Management, 12*, 231–240. doi:10.1089/pop.2009.0041

Harrison, P., & Lederberg, J. (Eds.). (1998). *Antimicrobial resistance: Issues and options. workshop report*. Washington, DC: National Academies Press.

Haynes, J. M. (2007). The ear as an alternative site for a pulse oximeter finger clip sensor. *Respiratory Care, 15*, 727–729.

Health Research Institute. (2012). *Medical cost trend: Behind the numbers 2013*. PricewaterhouseCoopers. Retrieved from http://www.uhc.com/live/uhc_com/Assets/Documents/PWC_MedicalCostTrend.pdf

Hendley, J. O. (1998). Epidemiology, pathogenesis, and treatment of the common cold. *Seminars in Pediatric Infectious Diseases, 9*, 50–55. doi.org/10.1016/S1045-1870(98)80051-4

Hicks, L. A. (2010, October). *Antimicrobial prescription data reveal wide geographic variability in antimicrobial use in the United States, 2009*. Presented at the 48th Annual Meeting of the Infectious Disease Society of America, Vancouver, Canada.

Hicks, L. A., Chien, Y., Taylor, T. H., Jr., Haber, M., & Klugman, K. P. (2011). Outpatient antibiotic prescribing and nonsusceptible *Streptococcus pneumoniae* in the United States, 1996-2003. *Clinical Infectious Diseases, 53*, 631–639. doi:10.1093/cid/cir443

Himes, J. H. (2009). Challenges of accurately measuring and using BMI and other indicators of obesity in children. *Pediatrics, 124*, S3–S22. doi:10.1542/peds.2008-3586D

Holmes, S., Mallet, S., & Peffers, S. (2009). PCRS-UK opinion sheet No. 28: Pulse oximetry in primary care. Retrieved from http://www.pcrs-uk.org/resources/os28_pulse_oximetry.pdf

Hooton, T. M. (2012, October 5). Acute complicated cystitis and pyelonephritis. *UpToDate*. Retrieved from http://www.uptodate.com/contents/acute-complicated-cystitis-and-pyelonephritis?source=search_result&search=Acute+complicated+cystitis+and+pyelonephritis&selectedTitle=1~49

Hooton, T. M., & Gupta, K. (2012, September 20). Urinary tract infections and asymptomatic bacteriuria in pregnancy. *UpToDate*. Retrieved from http://www.uptodate.com/contents/urinary-tract-infections-and-asymptomatic-bacteriuria-in-pregnancy?source=search_result&search=uti+pregnancy&selectedTitle=1~150

Hooton, T. M., & Stamm, W. E. (1997). Diagnosis and treatment of uncomplicated urinary tract infection. *Infectious Disease Clinics of North America, 11*, 551–581.

Howe, A. S., & Boden, B. P. (2007). Heat-related illness in athletes. *American Journal of Sports Medicine, 35*, 1384–1395.

Hwang, P., & Getz, A. (2012). Acute sinusitis and rhinosinusitis in adults: Treatment. *UpToDate*. Retrieved from http://www.uptodate.com/contents/acute-sinusitis-and-rhinosinusitis-in-adults-treatment

Institute for Clinical Systems Improvement (ICSI). (2006). *Uncomplicated urinary tract infection in women*. Bloomington, MN.

Institute for Clinical Systems Improvement (2011). *Healthcare guideline: Diagnosis and treatment of respiratory illness in children and adults* (3rd ed.). Retrieved July 04, 2012, from http://www.icsi.org/guidelines_and_more/gl_os_prot/respiratory_illness_in_children_and_adults_guideline_respiratory_illness_in_children_and_adults_guideline_13110.html

Institute of Medicine. (2000). *To err is human: Building a safer system.* Washington DC: National Academies Press.

Institute of Medicine. (2010, October 5). *The future of nursing: Leading change, advancing health.* Washington, DC: The National Academies Press. Retrieved from http://www.iom.edu/Reports/2010/The-Future-of-Nursing-Leading-Change-Advancing-Health.aspx

Jacobs, D. (2011, November 21). Evaluation of the red eye. *UpToDate.* Retrieved from http://www.uptodate.com/contents/evaluation-of-the-red-eye.

Jacobsen, L. M., & Antonellie, P. J. (2010). Errors in the diagnosis and management of necrotizing otitis externa. *Otolaryngology-Head and Neck Surgery, 143*, 506–509.

Jacoby, R., Crawford, A. G., Chaudhari, P., & Goldfarb, N. I. (2010). Quality of care for 2 common pediatric conditions treated by convenient care providers. *American Journal of Medical Quality, 26*, 53–58. doi:10.1177/1062860610375106

Juang, P. (2001). Red eye. In M. Bracker (Ed.), *The 5-minute sports medicine consult* (pp. 504–505). Philadelphia, PA: Lippincott Williams & Wilkins.

Kaplan, N. M., & Domino, F. J. Overview of hypertension in adults. *UpToDate.* Last updated June 26, 2012. Retrieved from http://www.uptodate.com/contents/overview-of-hypertension-in-adults

Kassel, J. C., King, D., & Spurling, G. K. (2010). Saline nasal irrigation for acute upper respiratory tract infections. *Cochrane Database of Systematic Reviews, 17*, CD006821. doi:10.1002/14651858.CD006821.pub2

Klein, R. (2012, January). Treatment of herpes simplex virus type 1 infection in immunocompetent patients. UpToDate. Retrieved from http://www.uptodate.com/contents/treatment-of-herpes-simplex-virus-type-1-infection-in-immunocompetent-patients?source=search_result&search=herpes+labialis&selectedTitle=1~57

Klein, J. O., & Pelton, S. (2012, August 1). Acute otitis media in children: Epidemiology, microbiology, clinical manifestations and complications. *UpToDate.* Retrieved December 20, 2011, from http://www.uptodate.com/contents/acute-otitis-media-in-children-epidemiology-microbiology-clinical-manifestations-and-complications?source=search_result&search=acute+otitis+media&selectedTitle=7~150

Kogutt, M., & Swischuk, L. E. (1973). Diagnosis of sinusitis in infants and children. *Pediatrics, 52*, 121–124.

Laryngitis. (2010, December 16). *PubMed Health.* Retrieved from http://www.ncbi.nlm.nih.gov/pubmedhealth/PMH0002361

Lewis, R. (2012, July 19). California pertussis epidemic reveal vaccine gap. *Medscape.* Retrieved from http://www.medscape.com/viewarticle/767702

Loeser, J. D., & Melzack, R. (1999). Pain: An overview. *Lancet, 353*, 1607–1609. doi:10.1016/S0140-6736(99)01311-2. doi:10.1016/S0140-6736(99)01311-2

Lu, P. J., & Nuorti, J. P. (2010) Pneumococcal polysaccharide vaccination among adults aged 65 years and older, United States, 1989-2008. *American Journal of Preventive Medicine, 39*, 287–295. doi:10.1016/j.amepre.2010.06.004

Luszczak, M. (2001). Evaluation and management of infants and young children with fever (Electronic version). *American Family Physician, 64*, 1219–1226.

Mackowiak, P. (1994). Fever: Blessing or curse? A unifying hypothesis (Electronic version). *Annals of Internal Medicine, 120*, 1037–1040.

Mahmood, A. R., & Narang, A. T. (2008.) Diagnosis and management of the acute red eye. *Emergency Medicine Clinics of North America, 26*, 35–55.

Malvey, D., & Fottler, M. D. (2006). The retail revolution in health care: Who will win and who will lose? *Health Care Management Review, 31*, 168–178.

Mandal, R., Patel, N., & Ferguson, B. J. (2012). Role of antibiotics in sinusitis. *Current Opinion Infectious Disease, 25*, 183–192.

Mandelco, B., & McCoy, J. K. (2012). Growth and development of the adolescent. In N. L. Potts & B. L. Mandelco (Eds.), *Pediatric nursing: Caring for children and their families* (3rd ed., 357–406). Clifton Park, NY: Delmar.

Mangione-Smith, R., Elliott, M. N., Stivers, T., McDonald, L. L., Heritage, J., & McGlynn, E. A. (2004). Racial/ethnic variation in parent expectations for antibiotics: Implications for public health campaigns. *Pediatrics, 113*, e385–e394.

Maron, B., Thompson, P. D., Ackerman, M. J., Balady, G., Berger, S., Cohen, D., & Puffer, J. C. (2007). Recommendations and considerations related to preparticipation screening for cardiovascular abnormalities in competitive athletes: 2007 update. *Circulation, 115*, 1643–1655. doi:10.1161/CIRCULATIONAHA.107.181423

May, A., & Bauchner, H. (1992). Fever phobia: The pediatrician's contribution (Electronic version). *Pediatrics, 90*, 851–854.

McCormick, D. P., Saeed, K. A., Pittman, C., Baldwin, C. D., Friedman, N., Teichgraeber, D. C., & Chonmaitree, T. (2003). Bullous myringitis: A case-control study. *Pediatrics, 112*, 982–986. doi:10.1542/peds.112.4.982

McCrory, D., & Lewis, S. Z. (2006). Methodology and grading of the evidence for diagnosis and management of cough: ACCP evidence. *Chest, 129*, 28S–32S.

Mehnert-Kay, S. A. (2005). Diagnosis and management of uncomplicated urinary tract infections. *American Family Physician, 72*(3), 451–456.

Mehrotra, A., & Lave, J. R. (2012). Visits to retail clinics grew fourfold from 2007 to 2009, although their share of overall outpatient visits remains low. *Health Affairs, 31*, 1–7. doi:10.1377/hlthaff.2011.1128

Mehrotra, A., Liu, H., Adams, J. L., Wang, M. C., Lave, J. R., Thygeson, M., & McGlynn, E. A. (2009). Comparing costs and quality of care at retail clinics with that of other medical settings for 3 common illnesses. *Annals of Internal Medicine, 151*, 321–328.

Mehrotra, A., Wang, M. C., Lave, J. R., Adams, J. L., & McGlynn, E. A. (2008). Retail clinics, primary care physicians, and emergency departments: A comparison of patients' visits. *Health Affairs, 27*, 1272–1282. doi:10.1377/hlthaff.27.5.1272

Meltzer, E. O., & Hamilos, D. L. (2011). Rhinosinusitis diagnosis and management for the clinician: A synopsis of recent concensus guidelines. *Mayo Clinic Proceedings, 86*, 427–443.

Meltzer, E. O., Hamilos, D. L., Hadley, J. A., Lanza, D. C., Marple, B. F., Nicklas, R. A., … Winther, B. (2006). Rhinosinusitis: Developing guidance for clinical trials. *The Journal of Allergy and Clinical Immunology, 118*(Suppl. 5), S17–S61. doi:10.1016/j.jaci.2006.09.005

Meltzer, E. O., Teper, A., & Danzig, M. (2008). Intranasal corticosteroids in the treatment of acute rhinosinusitis. *Current Allergy and Asthma Reports, 8*, 133–138.

Meneghetti, A. (2012, May 7). Upper respiratory tract infection. *Medscape*. Retrieved from http://emedicine.medscape.com/article/302460-overview

Mezey, M. D., McGivern, D. O., Sullivan-Marx, E. M., & Greenberg, S. A. (2003). *Nurse practitioners: Evolution of advanced practice* (4th ed.). New York, NY: Springer Publishing Company.

Michael, J. H., Hug, D., & Dowd, M. D. (2002). Management of corneal abrasion in children: A randomized clinical trial. *Annals of Emergency Medicine, 40*, 67–72.

Miller, J. L., & Silverstein, J. H. (2006). The metabolic syndrome: Growing challenge in primary care. *Contemporary Pediatrics, 23*, 32–45.

Mills, D., & Woodring, B. (2012). Growth and development of the toddler. In N. L. Potts & B. L. Mandelco (Eds.), *Pediatric nursing: Caring for children and their families* (3rd ed.,pp. 273–306). Clifton Park, NY: Delmar.

Mirza, S., & Richardson, H. (2005). Otic barotrauma from air travel. *The Journal of Laryngology and Otology, 119*, 366–370. doi:http://dx.doi.org/10.1258/0022215054273151

MN Community Measurement. (2010). 2011 Health care quality report. Retrieved from http://mncm.org/site/upload/files/2011HCQR3.30_FINAL.pdf

Mononucleosis. (2012, May 15). *PubMed Health.* Retrieved from http:///www.ncbi.nlm.nih.gov/pubmedhealth/PMH0001617/

Murphy, P., & Williams, S. (2010, June). National urgent care chart survey. *The Journal of Urgent Care Medicine.* Retrieved from http://jucm.com/pdf/2010%20JUCM%20Urgent%20Care%20Chart%20Research-1.pdf

National Cancer Institute. (2012). *Surveillance epidemiology and end results.* Retrieved from http://seer.cancer.gov/statfacts/html/testis.html

National Center for Complementary and Alternative Medicine. (2012, January 18). Colds/flu. Retrieved from http://nccam.nih.gov/health/flu

National Committee for Quality Assurance. (2011). *Continuous improvement and the expansion of quality measurement.* Retrieved from http://www.ncqa.org/Portals/0/Publications/Resource%20Library/SOHC/SOHC%202011-v2-web_2.22.12.pdf

National Committee for Quality Assurance. (2012). The state of health care quality, 2012. http://www.ncqa.org/tabid836/default.aspx

National Council on Patient Information and Education. (2004, April 1). Ten tips for parents. Retrieved from http://www.bemedwise.org/ten_ways/top_tips_parents.htm

National Heart, Lung, and Blood Institute. (2012). Assessing your weight and health risk. Retrieved from http://www.nhlbi.nih.gov/health/public/heart/obesity/lose_wt/risk.htm

National High Blood Pressure Education Program Working Group on Hypertension Control in Children and Adolescents. (1996). Update on the 1987 task force report on high blood pressure in children and adolescents: A working group report from the national high blood pressure education program. *Pediatrics, 98*(4 pt. 1), 649–658.

National Institutes of Allergy and Infectious Diseases. Sinusitis. Retrieved April 2012 from http://www.niaid.nih.gov/topics/sinusitis/Pages/Index.aspx

National Institute of Arthritis, Musculoskeletal and Skin Diseases. (2009, April). Sprains and strains. http://www.niams.nih.gov/Health_Info/Sprains_Strains/default.asp

Neilan, R. E., & Roland, P. S. (2010). Otalgia. *Medical Clinics of North America, 94*, 961–971.

Novak, E., & Allen, P. J. (2007). Prescribing medications in pediatrics: Concerns regarding FDA approval and pharmacokinetics. *Pediatric Nursing, 33*, 64–70.

O'Connor-Von, S. (2012). Growth and development of the school-age child. In N. L. Potts & B. L. Mandelco (Eds.), *Pediatric nursing: Caring for children and their families* (3rd ed., pp. 331–356). Clifton Park, NY: Delmar.

Organisation for Economic Co-Operation and Development (OECD). *OECD health data, 2012. How does the United States compare?* Retrieved from http://www.oecd.org/unitedstates/BriefingNoteUSA(2012).pdf

Palazzi, D. L. (2012, February 16). Approach to the child with fever of unknown origin. *UpToDate.* Retrieved from http://www.uptodate.com/contents/approach-to-the-child-with-fever-of-unknown-origin?source=search_results&search=approach+to+the+child+with+fever&selectedTitle=1~150

Palazzi, D. L., & Campbell, J. R. (2012, September 13). Acute cystitis in children older than two years and adolescents. *UpToDate.* Retrieved from http://www.uptodate.com/contents/acute-cystitis-in-children-older-than-two-years-and-adolescents?source=search_result&search=Acute+Cystitis+in+Children+Older+than+Two+Years+and+Adolescents&selectedTitle=1~150

Pichichero, M. E. (2012, September 13). Treatment and prevention of streptococcal tonsillopharyngitis. *UpToDate.* Retrieved from http://www.uptodate.com/contents/treatment-and-prevention-of-streptococcal-tonsillopharyngitis

Pleis, J. R., Lucas, J. W., & Ward, B. W. (2009). Summary health statistics for U.S. adults: National health interview survey 2008. *Vital and Health Statistics. Series 10, Data from the National Health Survey, 242,* 1–157. Retrieved from www.cdc.gov/nchs/data/series/sr_10/sr10_242.pdf

Pollack, C. E., & Armstrong, K. (2009). The geographic accessibility of retail clinics for underserved populations. *Archives of Internal Medicine, 169,* 945–949. doi:10.1001/archinternmed.2009.69

Prok, L., & McGovern, T. (2012, February 15). Poison ivy dermatitis. *UpToDate.* Retrieved from http://www.uptodate.com/contents/poison-ivy-toxicodendron-dermatitis?source=search_result&search=poison+ivy&selectedTitle=1~34

Ramakrishnan, K., Sparks, R. A., & Berryhill, W. E. (2007). Diagnosis and treatment of otitis media. *American Family Physician, 76,* 1650–1658.

Reeves, J. R. T., & Maibach, H. I. (1998). *Clinical dermatology illustrated: A regional approach* (3rd ed.). Philadelphia, PA: F. A. Davis Company.

Reid, R. O., Ashwood, J. S., Friedberg, M. W., Weber, E. S., Setodji, C. M., & Mehrotra, A. (2012). Retail clinic visits and receipt of primary care. *Journal of General Internal Medicine.* Published online ahead of print.

Reynolds, C. (2012). Growth and development of the preschooler. In N. L. Potts & B. L. Mandelco (Eds.), *Pediatric nursing: Caring for children and their families* (3rd ed. pp. 307–330). Clifton Park, NY: Delmar.

Rice, S. G. (2010). Medical conditions affecting sports participation. *Pediatrics, 121,* 841–848. doi:10.1542/peds.2008-0080

Richardson, M., & Lakhanpaul, M. (2007). Assessment and initial management of feverish illness in children younger than 5 years: Summary of NICE guidance (Electronic version). *British Medical Journal, 334,* 163–1164. doi:10.1136/bmj.39218.495255.AE

Royal College of Nursing. (2009). *The recognition and assessment of acute pain in children.* (Publication code: 003 542). Retrieved from http://www.rcn.org.uk/__data/assets/pdf_file/0004/269185/003542.pdf

Rudavsky, R., Pollack, C. E., & Mehrotra, A. (2009). The geographic distribution, ownership, prices, and scope of practice at retail clinics. *Annals of Internal Medicine, 151,* 315–320.

Rugwhani, N. (2011). Normal anatomic and physiologic changes with aging and related disease outcomes: A refresher. *Mount Sinai Journal of Medicine, 78,* 509–514. doi:10.1002/msj.20271

Scheid, D., & Hamm, R. M. (2004). Acute bacterial rhinosinusitis in adults: Part I. Evaluation. *American Family Physician, 70,* 1685–1692.

Schoenbaum, S. (1993). Feedback of clinical performance information. *HMO Practice/ HMO Group, 7,* 5–11.

Schmitt, B. (1980). Fever phobia: Misconception of parents about fever (Electronic version). *American Journal of Childhood Disease, 134,* 176–181.

Schwartz, B., Bell, D. M., & Hughes, J. M. (1997). Preventing the emergence of antimicrobial resistance. A call for action by clinicians, public health officials, and patients. *JAMA, 278,* 944–945. doi:10.1001/jama.1997.03550110082041

Schwartz, M. (Ed.). (2008). *Fever of unknown cause, pediatric.* Retrieved from http://www.5minuteconsult.com/5mc/20007322/fever-of-unknown-cause-pediatric-diagnosis

Scott, J. G., Cohen, D., DiCicco-Bloom, B., Orzano, A. J., Jaén, C. R., & Crabtree, B. F. (2001). Antibiotic use in acute respiratory infections and the ways patients pressure physicians for a prescription. *The Journal of Family Practice, 50,* 853–858.

Sethuraman, U., & Kamat, D. (2009). The red eye: Evaluation and management. *Clinical Pediatrics, 48*, 583–599. doi: 10.1177/0009922809333094

Sexton, D., & McClain, M. T. (2011, January 3). The common cold in adults: Diagnosis and clinical features. *UpToDate*. Retrieved from http://www.uptodate.com/contents/the-common-cold-in-adults-diagnosis-and-clinical-features?source=search_result&search=The+Common+cold+in+adults%3A+Diagnosis+and+clinical+features&selectedTitle=1~105

Shah, B. M., & Hajjar, E. R. (2012). Polypharmacy, adverse drug reactions and geriatric syndromes. *Clinical Geriatric Medicine, 28*, 173–186.

Shah, R. (2011, July 22). Acute laryngitis. *Medscape*. Retrieved from http://emedicine.medscape.com/article/864671-overview

Shah, S. (2012, May). Fever of unknown cause, pediatric. *5MinuteConsult*. Retrieved from http://www.5minuteconsult.com/5mc/20007322/fever-of-unknown-cause-pediatric-diagnosis

Shah, U. (2012, June 21). Tonsillitis and peritonsillar abscess. *Medscape*. Retrieved from http://emedicine.medscape.com/article/871977-overview

Shaikh, N., & Hoberman, A. (2012, August 29). Epidemiology and risk factors for urinary tract infections in children. *UpToDate*. Retrieved from http://www.uptodate.com/contents/epidemiology-and-risk-factors-for-urinary-tract-infections-in-children?source=search_results&search=epidemiology+and+risk+factors+for+urinary+tract+infections+in+children&selectedTitle=1~150

Shehab, N., Patel, P. R., Srinivasan, A., & Budnitz, D. S. (2008). Emergency department visits for antibiotic-associated adverse events. *Clinical Infectious Diseases, 47*, 735–743.

Sherman, J., & Sood, S. (2012). Current challenges in the diagnosis and management of fever (Electronic version). *Current Opinion in Pediatrics, 24*, 400–406.

Sheth, K. (2011, April 30). Anisocoria. *MedlinePlus*. Retrieved from http://www.nlm.nih.gov/medlineplus/ency/article/003314.htm

Shoup, J. (2011). Management of adult rhinosinusitis. *The Nurse Practitioner, 36*, 22–26. doi:10.1097/01.NPR.0000406485.59758.a8

Shulman, S. T., Bisno, A. L., Clegg, H. W., Gerber, M. A., Kaplan, E. L., Lee, G., & Van Beneden, C. (2012). Clinical practice guideline for the diagnosis and management of group A streptococcal pharyngitis: 2012 update by the infectious diseases society of America. *Clinical Infectious Diseases, 55*, e86–e102. doi:10.1093/cid/cis629

Simon, H. K. (2012, June 15). Pediatric pharyngitis. *UpToDate*. Retrieved from http://emedicine.medscape.com/article/967384-overview

Silvestri, R., & Weinberger, S. (2011, September 27). Evaluation of subacute and chronic cough in adults. *UpToDate*. Retrieved from http://www.uptodate.com/contents/evaluation-of-subacute-and-chronic-cough-in-adults?source=see_link

Small, C. B., Bachert, C., Lund, V. J., Moscatello, A., Nayak, A., & Berger, W. (2007). Judicious antibiotic use and intranasal corticosteroids in acute rhinosinusitis. *The American Journal of Medicine, 120*, 289–294.

Small, E. (2009). Preparticipation physical evaluation. In T. K. McInerny, H. M. Adam, D. E. Campbell, D. M. Kamat, & K. J. Kelleher (Eds.), *Textbook of pediatric care* (pp. 317–326). Elk Grove Village, IL: American Academy of Pediatrics.

Smetana, G. W. & Shmerling, R. H. (2002). Does this patient have temporal arteritis? *Journal of the American Medical Association, 287*(1):92–101. doi:10-1001/pubs.JAMA-ISSN-0098-7484-287-1-jrc10000

Spinks, A., Glasziou, P., & Del Mar, C. (2006). Antibiotics for sore throat. *Cochrane Database of Systematic Reviews, 4*. doi:10.1002/14651858.CD000023.pub3

Stead, W. Symptomatic treatment of acute pharyngitis in adults. *UpToDate*. Last modified May 21, 2012. Retrieved from http://www.uptodate.com/contents/symptomatic-treatment-of-acute-pharyngitis-in-adults

Stevens, V. J., Corrigan, S. A., Obarzanek, E., Bernauer, E., Cook, N. R., Hebert, P., … P. K. (1993). Weight loss intervention in phase 1 of the trials of hypertension prevention. *Archives of Internal Medicine, 153,* 849–858. doi:10.1001/archinte.1993.00410070039006

Stivers, T., Mangione-Smith, R., Elliott, M. N., McDonald, L., & Heritage, J. (2003). Why do physicians think parents expect antibiotics? What parents report vs what physicians believe. *The Journal of Family Practice, 52,* 140–148.

Strep throat—Topic overview. (2010, July 27). *WebMD.* Retrieved from http://www.webmd.com/oral-health/tc/strep-throat-topic-overview?print=true

Streptococcal pharyngitis. (2012, May 23). Retrieved from http://web.ebscohost.com/dynamed/detail?vid=3&hid=113&sid=06948a3e-5c77-4fb7-8866-11c9a24ff6c3%40sessionmgr115&bdata=JnNpdGU9ZHluYW1lZC1saXZlJnN jb3BlPXNpdGU%3d#db=dme&AN=115782

Subcommittee on Management of Acute Otitis Media. (2004). Diagnosis and management of acute otitis media. *Pediatrics, 113,* 1451–1465.

Sullivan, J., & Farrar, H. (2011). Clinical report—Fever and antipyretic use in children (Electronic version). *Pediatrics, 127,* 580–587. doi:10.1542/peds.2010-3852

Tarabishy, A. B., & Jeng, B. H. (2008). Bacterial conjunctivitis: A review for internists. *Cleveland Clinic Journal of Medicine, 75*(7), 507–512. doi:10.3949/ccjm.75.7.507

Terrie, Y. (2009, November 15). Cough and cold products. *Pharmacy times.* Retrieved from http://www.pharmacytimes.com/publications/issue/2009/november2009/OTCCoughCold-1109

Thygeson, M., Van Vorst, K. A., Maciosek, M. V., & Solberg, L. (2008). Use and costs of care in retail clinics versus traditional care sites. *Health Affairs, 27*(5):1283–1292. doi:10.1377/hlthaff.27.5.1283

Tyrrell, D. A. J., Cohen, S., & Schlarb, J. E. (1993). Signs and symptoms in common colds. *Epidemiology and Infection, 111,* 143–156. doi:http://dx.doi.org/10.1017/S0950268800056764

United States Department of Health and Human Services. (2010). *Healthy people 2010.* McLean, VA: International Medical Publishing, Inc.

United States Department of Justice Drug Enforcement Agency (2004, March). Steroids in today's world. Retrieved from http://www.deadiversion.usdoj.gov/pubs/brochures/steroids/professionals/index.html

United States Department of Health and Human Services. (2010). *Healthy people 2010.* McLean, VA: International Medical Publishing, Inc.

United States Department of Justice Drug Enforcement Agency. (2004). *Steroid abuse in today's society.* Retrieved from http://www.deadiversion.usdoj.gov/pubs/brochures/steroids/professionals/index.html

Uphold, C. R., & Graham, M. V. (2003). *Ocular foreign bodies.* Gainesville, FL: Barmarrae Books.

Uphold, C. R., & Graham, M. V. (Eds.). (2003a). Preparticipation sports examination. In *Clinical guidelines in child health* (3rd ed., pp. 44–51). Gainesville, FL: Barmarrae Books.

Uphold, C. R., & Graham, M. V. (Eds.). (2003b). *Clinical guidelines in family practice* (4th ed.). Gainesville, FL: Barmarrae Books.

VisionGain. (2010, July 15). *The-global-OTC-pharmaceutical-market-2010-2025.* Retrieved from http://www.visiongain.com/Report/500/The-Global-OTC-Pharmaceutical-Market-2010-2025

Vorvick, L. J. (2011, August 12). Physician assistant profession (PA). *MedlinePlus.* Retrieved from http://www.nlm.nih.gov/medlineplus/ency/article/001935.htm

Wald, E. (2012, June 12). Acute bacterial rhinosinusitis in children: Clinical features and diagnosis. *UpToDate.* Retrieved from http://www.uptodate.com/contents/acute-bacterial-rhinosinusitis-in-children-clinical-features-and-diagnosis

Wald, E. (2012, September 19). Approach to diagnosis of acute infectious pharyngitis in children and adolescents. *UpToDate*. Retrieved from http://www.uptodate.com/contents/approach-to-diagnosis-of-acute-infectious-pharyngitis-in-children-and-adolescents?source=see_link

Wang, M. C., Ryan, G., McGlynn, E. A., & Mehrotra, A. (2010). Why do patients seek care at retail clinics, and what alternatives did they consider? American Journal of Medical Quality, 25, 128–134. doi:10.1177/1062860609353201

Ward, M. A. (2012). Pathophysiology and management of fever in infants and children. *UpToDate*. Retrieved from http://www.uptodate.com/contents/pathophysiology-and-management-of-fever-in-infants-and-children?source=search_result&search=Pathophysiology+and+management+of+fever+in+infants+and+children&selectedTitle=1~150

Wedgbury, K., & Valler-Jones, T. (2008). Monitoring blood pressure using an automated sphygmomanometer. *British Journal of Nursing, 17*, 714–718.

Weinick, R. M., Burns, R. M., & Mehrotra, A. (2010). Many emergency department visits could be managed at urgent care centers and retail clinics. *Health Affairs, 29*, 1630–1636. doi:10.1377/hlthaff.2009.0748

Weinick, R. M., Pollack, C. E., Fisher, M. P., Gillen, E. M., & Mehrotra, A. (2010). Policy implications of the use of retail clinics. *RAND*. Retrieved from http://www.rand.org/pubs/technical_reports/TR810.html

Wenzel, R. P., & Fowler, A. A. (2006). Acute bronchitis. *New England Journal of Medicine, 355*, 2125–2130. doi:10.1056/NEJMcp061493

Weston, W., & Howe, W. (2011, August 26). Overview of dermatitis. *UpToDate*. Retrieved from http://www.uptodate.com/contents/overview-of-dermatitis?source=search_result&search=Overview+of+dermatitis&selectedTitle=1~150

White, B. (2011). Diagnosis and treatment of urinary tract infections in children. *American Family Physician, 83*, 409–415.

Woodburn, J. D., Smith, K. L., & Nelson, G. D. (2007). Quality of care in the retail health care setting using national clinical guidelines for acute pharyngitis. *American Journal of Medical Quality, 22*, 457–462. doi:10.1177/1062860607309626

World Health Organization. (2012). Immunization surveillance, assessment, and monitoring. Retrieved from www.who.int/immunization_monitor ing/en

Wu, F. (2012). Conjunctivitis. In F. Domino, R. Baldor, J. Golding, J. Grimes, & J. S. Taylor (Eds.), *The 5-minute clinical consult 2012* (20th ed., pp. 302–303). Philadelphia, PA: Lippencott, Williams, & Wilkins.

Wyant, C. (2008, July 29). BlueCross and BlueShield eliminates co-pays for retail customers. *Minneapolis/St. Paul Business Journal*. Retrieved from http://www.bizjournals.com/twincities/stories/2008/07/28/daily19.html

Zachary, K. C. Treatment of seasonal influenza in adults. *UpToDate*. Retrieved from http://www.uptodate.com/contents/treatment-of-seasonal-influenza-in-adults

Zorc, J. J., Kiddoo, D. A., & Shaw, K. N. (2005). Diagnosis and management of pediatric urinary tract infections. *Clinical Microbiology Reviews, 18*, 417–422. doi:10.1128/CMR.18.2.417-422.2005

Index

AAFP. *See* American Academy of Family Physicians
AAP. *See* American Academy of Pediatrics
ABRs. *See* acute bacterial rhinosinusitis
ACA. *See* Affordable Care Act
accessibility of clinics, convenient care model, 189
ACCP. *See* American College of Chest Physicians
Accreditation Commission for Health Care (ACHC), 195
accurate pulse oximetry, key factors in, 119
ACE inhibitors (ACE-Is), 64
acetaminophen, 48, 107, 108, 150
ACHC. *See* Accreditation Commission for Health Care
acute allergic contact dermatitis, treatment of, 86
acute bacterial otitis externa (AOE), 13
acute bacterial prostatitis, 78
acute bacterial rhinosinusitis (ABRs), 58
acute bronchitis, 65–66, 70, 156–158
acute closed-angle glaucoma, 33
acute dermatitis, 86
acute epididymitis, 78
acute otitis media (AOM), 13, 15–17, 158
acute pharyngitis, 158
acute pyelonephritis, 76
acute sinusitis (AS), 51, 158. *See also* sinusitis
  bacterial cause of, 52
  diagnosis of, 55, 56
  physical examination of, 53
acute urticaria, 89
adolescence, developmental stages/ physiologic changes of, 132

affordability, convenient care model, 187–189
Affordable Care Act (ACA), 9, 175, 177
Agency for Healthcare Research and Quality (AHRQ), 193
age-related changes for elderly patients, 134–135
age, respiratory rates by, 118
AHA. *See* American Heart Association
AHRQ. *See* Agency for Healthcare Research and Quality
AKS. *See* Anti-Kickback Statute
allergic conjunctivitis, 29
allergic contact dermatitis, 85–87
allergic rhinitis, 54
  shiners, 54
American Academy of Family Physicians (AAFP), 6, 8
American Academy of Pediatrics (AAP), 6, 8
American College of Chest Physicians (ACCP), 64
American Heart Association (AHA), 122
American Medical Association (AMA), 6
amoxicillin, 16, 45, 47
analgesics, 18
  OTC medications, 149–151
anaphylaxis, signs and symptoms of, 90
antibiotic ophthalmic treatment, 27
antibiotic resistance, 153, 156, 158
Antibiotic Resistance Monitoring in Ocular Microorganisms (ARMOR) study, 29
antibiotics, 16, 65, 70
antihistamines, 57, 68–69, 87
antihypertensives, 114

Anti-Kickback Statute (AKS), 203
antimicrobial treatment, sinusitis,
        58–59
antipyretic medications, use of,
        107, 108
antiviral agents, 93
AOM. *See* acute otitis media
Arizona regulations, 203
ARMOR study. *See* Antibiotic Resistance
        Monitoring in Ocular
        Microorganisms study
AS. *See* acute sinusitis
aspirin, 108, 151
asthma, 64
asymptomatic elevated BP, 113–114
asymptomatic low BP, 115
atopic dermatitis, 87–88
atrophic vaginitis, 79
augmentin, 16, 47
Aurora Health Care, 217
Aurora QuickCare Clinics, 217
azithromycin, 47

bacitracin, 85, 96
bacterial conjunctivitis, 28–29, 31
bacterial keratitis, 31
bacterial pharyngitis, 41, 43–46
bacterial sinusitis, 56–57, 158. *See also*
        sinusitis
balanitis, 78
balanoposthitis, 78
Baptist Express Care, 218
Baptist Health Systems, 218
Baptist Medical Center-Leake, 218
barotrauma, 18
bath oil, 88
beclomethasone, 69
Behçet's syndrome, dysuria, 79
Bellin Health, 218–219
Best Pharmaceuticals for Children Act,
        132–133
bicillin, 47
blepharitis, 36
blisters, 96
blood pressure (BP), 111–112
        adults, JNC 7—classification of, 115
        definitions and etiologies of, 112–113
        elevated, 113–115
body temperature, fluctuations in, 117
BP. *See* blood pressure

bradycardia, 116
bronchitis, 65–66
        acute, 156–158
        in retail-based clinics, 154
bullous impetigo, 92
bullous myringitis, 18
burns, 95–97

CAMAC. *See* Comprehensive
        Accreditation Manual for
        Ambulatory Care
capillary refill time, 104
cardiac auscultation, 123
Careworks, 220
CCA. *See* Convenient Care Association
CCI. *See* convenient care industry
CDC. *See* Centers for Disease Control and
        Prevention
cellulitis, 20, 95
Centene Corporation, 225
Centers for Disease Control and
        Prevention (CDC), 138, 140
        Get Smart: Know When
                Antibiotics Work program, 155,
                156, 158–159
        resources of, 141
Centor score for RST, 42
cerumen impaction, 18–19
cerumenolytics, 18–19
cervicitis, 78
CFU. *See* colony-forming unit
chalazion, 34–35
chest cold, 67
chondritis, 20
chronic allergic contact dermatitis, 86
chronic prostatitis, 78
chronic urticaria, 89
CLIA. *See* Clinical Laboratory
        Improvement Act
clinical advisory board, 8
clinical decision support, 159
Clinical Laboratory Improvement Act
        (CLIA), 5
        waived test, 27
clinical pearls for antibiotic avoidance,
        156–158
clinic operators, profiles of
        Aurora QuickCare Clinics, 217
        Baptist Express Care, 218
        Baptist Health Systems, 218

Bellin Health, 218–219
Geisinger Careworks, 219–220
Harrison Memorial Hospital, 220
HealthCaring Clinic, 220–221
Heritage Valley Health System, 221
Lakeview Health//Stillwater Medical
    Group, 221–222
Lindora Health Clinics, 222–223
Little Clinic health care clinics,
    223–224
MEDPOINT express, 224
MHSI, 225
MinuteClinic, 225–226
North Mississippi Health Services,
    226–227
RediClinic, 227
Sutter Express Care, 229
Take Care Health Systems, 227–228
Target Clinic, 228–229
colony-forming unit (CFU), 77
combination therapy, 114
common cold, 64–65, 70, 148, 158
    OTC medications, 147–149
common family illnesses, treatment for,
    217, 229
communication of OTC medications,
    146–147
community-based health care, 221
community pharmacy, 222
Comprehensive Accreditation Manual for
    Ambulatory Care (CAMAC), 195
conflict-of-interest argument, 6
conjunctivitis
    allergic, 29
    bacterial, 28–29, 31
    for contact lens wearers, 32
    subconjunctival hemorrhage, 29–30
    viral, 26–27
contact dermatitis, 85
contact lens
    related infectious keratitis, 32
    wearers, eye infections for, 29, 32
Convenient Care Association (CCA), 5–6,
    195–196
convenient care clinics (CCCs)
    co-branded, 162
    developmental stages/physiologic
        changes
        adolescence (12 to 18 years), 132
        infant to 12 months, 130
        preschool (3 to 6 years), 131

school (6 to 12 years), 131–132
toddler (12 to 36 months),
    130–131
dollars and cents of running, 179–186
elderly patients, 133–135
geriatrics, 133–135
leadership, 159, 168
long-term considerations, 133
management, strategies for, 158–159
marketing, focus on multiple target
    audiences, 166–168
model, retail-based, 3–7
pediatrics, 129, 132–133
physical space of, 164
physiological changes, 134–135
providers, strategies for, 154–156
retail, 161–169
strategies to improve antibiotic
    prescribing in, 153–159
    clinical pearls for antibiotic
        avoidance, 156–158
    clinic management strategies,
        158–159
    future of, 159
    in retail-based clinics, 154
    strategies to encourage, 154–155
convenient care industry (CCI), 218, 223,
    229
    founding of, 5–6
    future directions of, 8–9
    history of, 1–2
    nonphysician providers role in primary
        care, 2–3
    quality and safety standards for,
        7–8
convenient care setting, collaboration and
    partnership in
    CCCs, 205
    fraud and abuse considerations,
        203–204
    NPs, 202–203
    PAs, 203
    PCP, establishing relationships with,
        204–205
    practice and derived medical authority,
        scope of, 201–202
convenient medical services, 224
conventional health care delivery
    system, 2
corneal abrasions, 30–31
corneal epithelial defects, 32

cornea, staining of, 24–25
corticosteroids, 48–49
Corynebacterium diphtheria, 43
cough
  case study for, 61, 63
  differential diagnosis of
    infectious, 64–67
    noninfectious, 64
  disposition of, 70–71
  OTC medications, 147–149
  pathophysiology and epidemiology of,
    61–62
  patient approach with, 62–63
  red flags for, 63
  suppressants, 68
  treatment of
    managing expectations and patient
     education, 67
    symptomatic care, 67–69
    targeted therapy, 69–70
cromolyn sodium (intranasal), 70
customer satisfaction, measuring,
  171–178
CVS Caremark Corporation, 6, 225

DASH diet, 114
dental abscess, 54
dental disease, 21
dermatitis. *See* eczema
dermatology for OTC medications,
  149
dermatomal distribution, herpes zoster
  in, 94
dermatophytes, 97
dexamethasone, 48
dextromethorphan for nonproductive
  cough, 149
diagnostic testing, 77
disruptive innovation, CCCs as, 1,
  208–209
dizziness, 113
dosage forms for topical therapy,
  150
doxycycline, 58
dysfunctional elimination, 79
dysuria
  infectious differential diagnosis of,
    78
  noninfectious differential diagnosis of,
    78–79

ear
  canal, cleaning debris from, 14
  discharge, 12, 13, 19
  examination, 21
ear, nose and throat (ENT) specialist, 12
ear pain
  case study, 11
  clinical evaluation, 12
  differential diagnosis
    AOM, 13, 15–17
    bullous myringitis, 18
    cerumen and cerumen impaction,
     18–19
    ETD, 17
    OME, 17
    primary otalgia, 13–15
    TM rupture, 18
  due to dental processes, 13
  physical examination, 12–13
  primary ear infections, 19–22
eczema
  allergic contact dermatitis, 85–87
  atopic dermatitis, 87–88
  contact dermatitis, 85
  herpes simplex (HSV-1), 93
  impetigo, 92–93
  irritant-contact dermatitis, 87
  scabies, 90–92
  seborrheic dermatitis, 88
  urticaria (hives), 88–90
electronic health records (EHRs), 4, 159,
  165, 190, 196–198, 214
electronic medical records (EMRs),
  184, 214
electronic self-registration kiosks, 184
empirical treatment for pharyngitis, 46–47
empiric antimicrobial therapy of ABRS, 58
empiric monotherapy of ABRS, 58
EMRs. *See* electronic medical records
Enterobacteriaceae, 77
ENT specialist. *See* ear, nose and throat
  specialist
epiglottitis, 40
Epstein–Barr virus, 45
erythromycin, 28, 47
Escherichia coli, 74
ETD. *See* eustachian tube dysfunction
Ethics in Patient Referrals Act, 203
eustachian tube dysfunction (ETD), 17
evidence-based guidelines, CCC, 198
eyelid swelling, 29, 34–36

False Claims Act, 203
family illnesses
    medication for, 229
    treatment for, 217
FastCare retail health clinic model, 219
FBs. *See* foreign bodies
federally qualified health center (FQHC),
    225
fever, 53, 54, 56, 65
    adults with, 109
    approaches
        assessment of, 101–102
        illness history/systems review,
            102–103
        physical examination of, 103–104
    case study for, 99–100
    CCC approach, 101
    common causes of, 105
    defined, 99
    diagnosis of
        differential, 105
        follow-up, 108–109
        referrals, 109
        testing, 106–107
    management, 108
    parameters for, 100
    treatment, 107–108
fever phobia, 101, 108
first-generation H1 antihistamines, 89
fluorescein staining, 24–25, 30–32
fluoroquinolones, 20
flu shots, 137
fluticasone, 69
foreign bodies (FBs), 20
    of conjunctiva, 31
    sensation of, 24–25, 27
FQHC. *See* federally qualified health
    center
fungal infections, 97
future of CCCs
    disruptive innovation theory, 207–209
    expanding service offerings, 210
    growth pathway, 212–213
    professionals in, 211
    strategic questions, industry, 209
    value of convenience, 212

GABHS. *See* Group A β-hemolytic
    streptococcus
GAS. *See* Group A streptococcus

gastroesophageal reflux disease
    (GERD), 64
Geisinger Careworks, 219–220
Geisinger Health System, 219, 220
GERD. *See* gastroesophageal reflux
    disease
Get Smart: Know When Antibiotics Work
    program, 155, 156, 158–159
glucocorticoids
    benefits, 57
    brief course of, 89
    topical, 14, 69
gross hearing test, 12
Group A β-hemolytic streptococcus
    (GABHS)
    pharyngitis, 39, 41–47
Group A streptococcus (GAS), 158
growth spurt, 132

Haemophilus influenzae, 58
Harrison Memorial Hospital, 220
head tumor, 22
health care delivery
    models, 225–226
    systems, 9
Healthcare Effectiveness and Data
    Information Set (HEDIS),
    194–195, 197
health care providers
    misconceptions to provide vaccina-
        tions, 138
    to promote health by vaccination,
        138–139
    vaccine recommendations of, 141
health care quality, certification and
    accreditation of, 195
health care reform, future of
    access, payment and patient communi-
        cation, 214–215
    integrated EMRs, 214
    nursing practice and licensure scope
        expansion, 213–214
health care services, 218
health care standards, 194
health care system
    CCCs, 212–213
    integrated, 217
HealthCaring Clinic, 220–221
HealthCaring Company, 220
health education opportunity, PPEs, 124–125

Health Insurance Portability and
    Accountability Act, 8, 122
health systems
    increased involvement of, 7
    and payers, partnership opportunities
        with, 224
Healthy People 2010, and vaccination
    targets, 138
Healthy People 2020, and vaccination
    targets, 141
hearing impairment, 12
heart murmur, 123
heart rate, 111, 116, 131, 134
HEDIS. *See* Healthcare Effectiveness and
    Data Information Set
hematuria, 74, 77
"herd immunity," 138
Heritage Valley Health System, 221
herpes simplex (HSV-1), 32–33, 93
herpes simplex encephalitis, clinical
    symptoms of, 104
herpes zoster (shingles), 93–94
    burn, 95–97
    cellulitis, 95
    tinea (fungal infections), 97
herpes zoster oticus, 20
herpetic keratitis, 32
herpetiform lesions, 84
hives, 88–90
honey, diminishing cough, 68
hordeolum, 35
HSV-1. *See* herpes simplex
hypertension, 123
    for adults in United States, 111–112
    and BP, 112
    in children and adolescents, 115–116
    diagnosis of, 115
    in elderly, 134
    sign of uncontrolled, 30
    treatment of, 114, 115
hypertensive emergency, defined, 113
hypertensive urgency, defined, 113
hyperthermia, 101, 117
hyphema, 26, 33, 34
hypopyon, 26, 30, 31, 33
hypotension, 112, 113, 115
hypothermia, 117

ibuprofen, 48, 70, 80, 107, 108, 117, 150
immune system, elderly patients, 134

immunizations, 137, 139
    barriers, 138–139
    of children and adults, 137, 141
    records of, 139
impetigo, 92–93
induration, skin, 84
infectious differential diagnosis, 64–67
    of dysuria in males and females, 78
inflammation, 61–62
influenza, 66, 69–70
    pharyngitis caused by, 45
    vaccine, 137
infrastructure-independent services,
    211
Institute of Medicine and National
    Quality Forum, 204
Institute of Medicine's Committee on the
    Future of Primary Care, 2
in-store clinics, 223, 227
insurance-based primary care provider,
    169
integrated electronic medical records,
    214
interstitial cystitis, 79
intranasal steroids, 57
ipratropium, 69, 70
iritis, 25, 33
irritant-contact dermatitis, 87
irritants, 78–79
itch, 87–88

Jefferson School of Population Health
    (JSPH), 195
jet-powered canal irrigators, 19
JNC 7 guidelines, 115
Joint Commission on Accreditation of
    Hospitals (JCAHO), 195

Kawasaki disease, clinical symptoms of,
    104
keratitis
    bacterial, 31
    contact lens–related infectious, 32
    herpetic, 32
kidneys
    age-related changes, 134
    stones, 74, 76, 77
"kissing disease." *See* mononucleosis
Kroger Company, 224

labial adhesions, 79
Lakeview Health/Stillwater Medical
    Group, 221–222
laryngitis, 45
larynx, 22, 45
leadership, CCC, 159
Lean for Life® program, 223
lesion type, 83, 84
leukocyte esterase test, 77
levofloxacin, 58
licensed practical nurses (LPNs), 202
lichenification, 84
lightheadedness, 89, 113
Lindora Health Clinics, 222–223
linear lesions, 84
Little Clinic, 223–224
liver, age-related changes, 134
low BP emergencies, 113
low-potency topical corticosteroid, 88
lozenges, 48, 49, 68
LPNs. *See* licensed practical nurses

macrolides, 16, 58
malignant external otitis, 14–15
Managed Health Services, 225
Marfan syndrome, 123
mastoiditis, 19
medical authority, practice and derived,
    201–202
medical community, target audiences,
    166–167
medical establishment, initial challenges
    from, 6
medication for family illnesses, 229
MEDPOINT express, 224
Memorial Health System, 224
meningitis, 103, 105
    clinical symptoms of, 104
meningococcal disease, clinical symptoms
    of, 104
Midtown Piggly Wiggly, 225
Milwaukee Health Services, Inc. (MHSI),
    225
Minnesota health plan, 154
minor illnesses, treatment of, 218
MinuteClinic, 2, 3, 6, 225–226
Mississippi Hospital for Restorative Care,
    218
mononucleosis, 45, 106, 107
monospot test, 45

monotherapy, primary drugs used in, 114
moxifloxacin, 58
musculoskeletal examination, two-
    minute, 123–124
Mycoplasma pneumonia, 43, 69
mycoplasmic lower respiratory tract
    infections, 67

nasal decongestion, 148
nasal foreign body, 54
nasal sprays for common cold, 148
National Committee for Quality
    Assurance (NCQA), 195
National Quality Measures Clearinghouse
    (NQMC), 193–194
neck tumors, 22
necrotizing OE, 14
Neisseria gonorrhoeae, 29, 43
nickel dermatitis, 86
nitrates, UTI, 77
NMHS. *See* North Mississippi Health
    Services
nocturia, 74
nonbullous impetigo, 92
non-Group A streptococcus, 49
nonherpetic viral conjunctivitis, 27
noninfectious differential diagnosis
    of cough, 64
    of dysuria, 78–79
nonphysician providers in primary care,
    2–3
nonprescription medication, 144
nonsteroidal anti-inflammatory drugs
    (NSAIDs), 14, 17, 48, 68, 150
nonsuppurative complication, 46
North Mississippi Health Services
    (NMHS), 226–227
NPs. *See* nurse practitioners
NQMC. *See* National Quality Measures
    Clearinghouse
NSAIDs. *See* nonsteroidal anti-inflamma-
    tory drugs
nummular lesions, 84, 97
nurse practitioners (NPs), 2, 197, 202–203
    expanded scope of, 213–214
    MHS CCC, 225
    perform physical examinations and
        treat common illnesses, 224
    role of, 227–228
    in telehealth context, 210

nursing
    expanded scope of, 213–214
    and leadership, 227, 228

obesity, children, 133
OE. *See* otitis externa
Office of Disease Prevention and Health
    Promotion, 137
OME. *See* otitis media with effusion
online preregistration kiosks, 184
onychomycosis infections, 97
ophthalmology, 23, 26, 29, 32–34
oral steroids, 86
orbital cellulitis, 35, 53
orthostatic hypotension, 113
osteomyelitis, clinical symptoms
    of, 104
otalgia, 11
    primary, 13–15
    secondary, 21–22
otitis externa (OE), 12–15
otitis media, 13, 16, 106, 107
otitis media with effusion (OME), 17
otoscopic examination for ear, 12, 15
outpatient surgery centers, 223
over-the-counter (OTC) medications,
    68, 143
    analgesics, 149–151
    background, 144–145
    communication, 146–147
    cough and cold, 147–149
    dermatology, 149
    patient information for, 145–146

pain medication, 93, 94
pain, sinus, 53, 57
parotitis, 22
partial thickness burns (second degree),
    95
PAs. *See* physician assistants
patient-centered medicine, 222
patient-centric practices, 8
patient-driven performance standards,
    7–8
patients
    approach with urinary complaints,
        74–76
    chief complaints from, 52
    convenient access for, 219

education, 59–60
    information for OTC medications,
        145–146
    low-cost access point for, 224
    misconceptions, barriers to immuniza-
        tions, 138–139
    red flag warnings for, 53
    satisfaction for health care service,
        168–169
    take-home points for, 80–81
    vital signs. *See* vital signs, patients
PCP. *See* primary care physician
Pediatric Research Equity Act in 2003,
    132–133
pediatrics
    CCC setting, 129
    patient, chronic diseases in, 133
peer review, 198–199
pelvic inflammatory disease, 78
penicillin, 58
penicillin G, 47
penicillin V, 47
penlight examination, eye, 25, 30, 32
peritonsillar abscess (PTA), 40, 41
pertussis, 69
pharmacotherapy for mild-to-moderate
    pain, 150
pharyngitis, 21, 39, 106, 107, 158
    caused by influenza, 45
    diagnosis, 41–43
    differential diagnosis, 43–46
    patient education, 49
    symptoms and clinical emergencies, 40–41
    treatment, 46–49
pharynx, lesions of, 21
phenylephrine, OTC medications, 148
physician assistants (PAs), 2, 197, 203, 225
physician-based care models, 191
planogram, 140
PMNs. *See* polymorphonuclear cells
pneumococcal vaccine in adults, 138
pneumonia, 66, 104
pneumotoscopy, 12
point-of-care (POC) tests, 106
polymorphonuclear cells (PMNs), 62
postnasal drip. *See* upper airway cough
    syndrome (UACS)
poststreptococcal glomerulonephritis, 46
PPEs. *See* preparticipation physical
    evaluations
pregnancy, 81

preparticipation physical evaluations
(PPEs), 121
administration, 122
clearance for participation, 125–127
health education opportunity, 124–125
history, 122–123
physical examination, 123–124
referral for, 127
preschool children, health care providers,
131
prescription medication, 144, 148
prescriptive authority, 202
preseptal cellulitis, 35
primary care
changes in nature of satisfaction with,
174–177
current state of satisfaction with,
171–174
delivery models
disruption of, 211
traditional, service offerings
expansion, 210
delivery venues, disruptive innovation
in, 209
nonphysician providers in, 2–3
satisfaction with, 177–178
primary care physician (PCP), 171,
175–177, 188, 189, 191, 204–205
primary care provider. See primary care
physician (PCP)
primary otalgia, 13–15
profit and loss (P&L) statement of sample
CCC, 180–183
provider satisfaction for health care
service, 168–169
pseudoephedrine, OTC medications,
148
Pseudomonas, 32
Pseudomonas aeruginosa, 29
PTA. See peritonsillar abscess
public skepticism, 6
pulse oximetry, 118–119
pushing fluids, 108
pyelonephritis, 82

quality assurance of CCI, 8
quality health services, 218, 219
quality metrics, 193–194
recertification, 196
at TCHS, 197–198

quality of care, 6
commitment to, 7–8
convenient care model, 190–191
evidence of, 196–199
retail clinic, 165–166, 168–169
quality standards for industry,
establishment of, 7
QuickMedx, 2, 3, 6

Ramsay Hunt syndrome, 20
RAND study, 179
rapid strep test (RST), 41–43, 49
rashes
description of, 83
diagnosing, 83
eczema. See eczema
varicella/herpes zoster (shingles),
93–97
recurrent infections, 82
red eye
case study, 23, 26
conditions required for warrant
referral, 31–34
conjunctivitis. See conjunctivitis
differential diagnosis, 34–36
fluorescein staining, 24–25
patient history, 23–25
physical examination, 25–26
red flags, 25–26
symptoms, 26–31
red flags, 63
ENT, 13, 15
eye, 25–26
for patient, 53, 60
of UTIs, 76
RediClinic, 184, 227
registered nurses (RNs), 202
respiration, 118–119
respiratory fluoroquinolone (levo-
floxacin/moxifloxacin), 58
respiratory infections, antibiotics for,
156–158
respiratory rates by age, 118
retail-based convenient care clinic model
accessibility, 189
affordability, 187–189
antibiotic prescribing in, 154
clinic marketing, 166–168
clinic operations, 164–166
construction phase of, 166

retail-based convenient care clinic
    model (*cont.*)
  description, 3–5
  evaluation, operational measures, and
    quality of care, 168–169
  future directions of, 8–9
  increased involvement of health
    systems, 7
  initial challenges, 6
  as part of larger network, 169
  quality care, 190–191
  selecting retail partner. *See* retail part-
    ner, selecting
retail partner, selecting
  design and construction, 163–164
  location, 162–163
  negotiating lease, 163
reticulated lesions, 84
retropharyngeal abscess, 40–41
Reye's syndrome, 48
rhinosinusitis. *See* sinusitis
rhinovirus, 45
Rite Aid, 223
RNs. *See* registered nurses
RST. *See* rapid strep test

safety standards for industry, 7–8
saline irrigation, 57
Sarcoptes scabiei var. *hominis*, 90–91
scabies, 90–92
scarlatiniform rash, 44
scarlet fever, 44
seborrheic dermatitis, 88
secondary otalgia, 21–22
septic arthritis, clinical symptoms
    of, 104
sexual activity, UTIs, 74
shingles. *See* herpes zoster
short-course antibiotic therapy, 79
silver sulfadiazine, 96–97
sinusitis
  acute. *See* acute sinusitis
  bacterial, 55–57, 158
  case study for, 51, 55
  definitions and pathophysiology of,
    51–52
  diagnoses, 54–55
  infectious disease society of America,
    guidelines for, 55, 56
  markers for, 55

  patient education of, 59–60
  recommended antibiotics of, 59
  red flags in history/examination, 53
  symptoms, 52–55
  treatment of, 57–59
  viral, 55–57
sinus pain, 53
SMG. *See* Stillwater Medical Group
Snellen visual acuity test, 25
sore throat, 158
  case study, 39
  patient education, 49
  pharyngitis. *See* pharyngitis
spectrophotometric device, 118
sports physicals, 121–127
sputum, 65
staffing, retail clinic, 165
Stark Law, 203
steroids, 86, 87, 94
Stillwater Medical Group (SMG), 222
store personnel, target audiences, 167
strep pharyngitis, 44
Streptococcus pneumoniae, 58
subacute allergic contact dermatitis, 86
subconjunctival hemorrhage, 29–30
superficial burns (first degree), 95
suppurative complications, 44, 46
Sutter Express Care clinics, 229
SVR. *See* systemic vascular resistance
swimmers ear. *See* acute bacterial otitis
    externa
symptomatic treatment, 57
systemic therapy for pharyngitis, 48
systemic vascular resistance (SVR),
    104

tachycardia, 116
Take Care Clinics, 227–228
Take Care Health Systems (TCHS), 197,
    198, 227–228
target audiences, 166–168
Target Clinic, 228–229
targeted therapy, 69–70
target (or bull's-eye) lesions, 84
TCHS. *See* Take Care Health Systems
temperature abnormalities, 117
temporal arteritis, 21–22
temporomandibular joints (TMJs)
    dysfunction, 12, 21
tetanus prophylaxis, 97

The Joint Commission, 195
third-generation oral cephalosporin plus
    clindamycin, 58
third-party payers, 184
throat sprays for sore throat, 48
throat swab technique, 42
tinea (fungal infections), 97
TM. *See* tympanic membrane
TMJs dysfunction. *See* temporomandibu-
    lar joints dysfunction
tonsillitis of pharynx, 21
topical corticosteroid, 88, 97
topical decongestants, 68
topical medications, 93
topical saline, 68
topical steroids, 86, 87
topical therapy, 92
    dosage forms of, 150
    for pharyngitis, 48
Traffic Light System for risk assessment,
    101, 102
training, retail clinic, 165
transillumination, 53
trauma, 31, 79
Trichophyton rubrum, 97
Trichophyton tonsurans, 97
trimethoprim-sulfamethoxazole, 58
two-minute musculoskeletal examination,
    123–124
tympanic membrane (TM), 11, 13–15, 158
    rupture of, 18
    spontaneous rupture of, 19

UACS. *See* upper airway cough
    syndrome
upper airway cough syndrome (UACS),
    64
upper respiratory tract infections (URIs),
    45–46, 54, 56
    case study for, 61, 63
    patient care with, 62
    treatment of, 67–70
urethral strictures, 79
urethritis, 78
urinary stones, 79
urinary tract infections (UTIs), 106
    case study for, 73
    clinical symptoms of, 104
    diagnosis and differential diagnosis of,
        77–79

disposition and patient education of,
    80–81
epidemiology and pathophysiology of,
    73–74
patient approach with, 74–76
special considerations of, 81–82
treatment of, 79–80
typical symptoms of, 75–76
urine culture, 77
urine dipstick, 77
URIs. *See* upper respiratory tract
    infections
urticaria (hives), 88–90
U.S. Health System, 172–174
Utilization Review Accreditation
    Commission, 195
UTIs. *See* urinary tract infections

vaccinations, 137–141
    documentation of, 139
    error or adverse reaction, 140–141
    for promoting health, 138–139
    providing, 139–140
    rates, 137–138
    resources for health care professionals,
        141
Vaccine Adverse Event Reporting System,
    140
Vaccine Information Statement (VIS),
    139
vaccine-preventable disease rates in
    United States, 138
vaginitis, 78
varicella, 93–97
ventilation tubes for ear infections, 12
verrucous lesions, 84
viral conjunctivitis, 26–27
viral infections, 158
viral pharyngitis, 45
viral sinusitis, 52, 56. *See also* sinusitis
VIS. *See* Vaccine Information
    Statement
visit records of CCCs, 4–5
vital signs, patients
    body temperature, 117
    BP, 111–115
    heart rate, 116
    hypertension in children and
        adolescents, 115–116
    hypotension, 115

vital signs, patients (*cont.*)
    respiration, 118–119
vocal folds, swelling and erythema of, 45

Walgreens, 227, 228
Weigh Forward program, 227
weight loss, 114
wheezing, 66

white coat hypertension concept,
    112
written protocols, 203

xanthoma, 84

zosteriform lesions, 84